TOPICS IN HEART FAILURE MANAGEMENT

Edited by **Giuseppe Rescigno**
and **Michael S. Firstenberg**

Topics in Heart Failure Management
http://dx.doi.org/10.5772/intechopen.74704
Edited by Giuseppe Rescigno and Michael S. Firstenberg

Contributors

Massimo Baraldo, Sandro Sponga, Ugolino Livi, Okechukwu Ogah, Karen Sliwa, Adewole Adebiyi, Emmanuel Andres, Oleksii Korzh, Chih-Hsin Hsu, Wei-Ting Li, Giuseppe Rescigno

First published in London, United Kingdom, 2019 by IntechOpen
IntechOpen is the global imprint of INTECHOPEN LIMITED, registered in England and Wales, registration number: 11086078, The Shard, 25th floor, 32 London Bridge Street
London, SE19SG – United Kingdom
Printed in Croatia

British Library Cataloguing-in-Publication Data
A catalogue record for this book is available from the British Library

Additional hard and PDF copies can be obtained from orders@intechopen.com

Topics in Heart Failure Management, Edited by Giuseppe Rescigno and Michael S. Firstenberg
p. cm.
Print ISBN 978-1-83880-947-8
Online ISBN 978-1-83880-948-5
eBook (PDF) ISBN 978-1-83880-949-2

For EU product safety concerns:
IN TECH d.o.o., Prolaz Marije Krucifikse Kozulić 3, 51000 Rijeka, Croatia,
info@intechopen.com or visit our website at intechopen.com.

Meet the editors

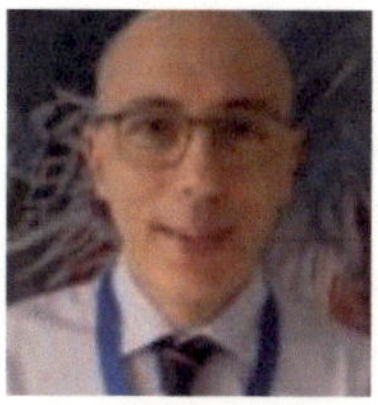

Mr. Giuseppe Rescigno graduated in Pavia, Italy, where he completed his general surgery training. He then moved to France to become a cardiac surgeon for adults. On his return to Italy, he worked in several hospitals. He is currently a member of the surgical team of the Royal Wolverhampton NHS Trust in Wolverhampton, UK. Clinical research has always been one of his main activities. He has published more than 50 articles in peer-reviewed journals. He was investigator surgeon of the STICH (Surgical Treatment for Ischemic Heart Failure) trial in Bergamo. In 2001–2002, he was lecturer for a PhD course at the University of Modena (Italy). He holds one patent on an original technique to assess bronchial ischemia after lung transplantation.

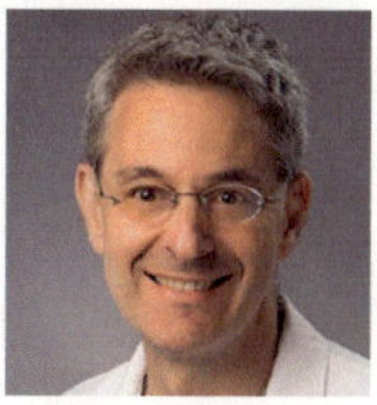

Dr. Michael S. Firstenberg is a board-certified thoracic surgeon practicing adult cardiac surgery at the Medical Center of Aurora (Colorado, USA) where he serves as the chief of cardiothoracic and vascular surgery. He currently holds adjunct appointments in the Colleges of Medicine and Graduate Studies at Northeast Ohio Medical University and serves on the teaching faculty at the Rocky Vista University. He attended Case Western Reserve University Medical School, received his general surgery training at University Hospitals in Cleveland, and completed a fellowship in thoracic surgery at the Ohio State University. He also obtained advanced training in heart failure surgical therapies at the Cleveland Clinic. He is an active member of the Society of Thoracic Surgeons, American Association of Thoracic Surgeons, American College of Cardiology, and American College of Academic International Medicine (for which he is a founding fellow). He currently serves as chair of the American College of Cardiology Credentialing and Member Services Committee as well as is active on several other national society committees. He is the author of well over 200 peer-reviewed manuscripts, abstracts, and book chapters. He has edited several textbooks on topics ranging from medical leadership, patient safety, endocarditis, and extracorporeal membrane oxygenation—all of which include topics on which he has lectured worldwide.

Contents

Preface

Without a doubt, both acute and chronic heart failure are major clinical and healthcare problems. The number of patients with some form of heart failure will continue to increase despite advances in therapies—a fact that is true worldwide. Furthermore, patient expectations are also increasing with regard to advances in all forms of therapy. Fortunately, progress in drug therapy, surgical and catheter-based options, along with mechanical circulation assist devices and transplantation, is now able to offer an improved quality of life for years after an initial diagnosis of heart failure. However, the paradox is that patients are becoming more complex and frequently a multidisciplinary team approach is necessary for optimal management with multiple objectives, including quality and quantity of life, reduced hospitalizations and healthcare costs, and a recognition of the role of appropriate referral to a hospice and palliative care when further care might be approaching futility. The aim of this book is to gather different perspectives from highly esteemed clinicians and researchers on a variety of topics pertaining to the management of patients with some form of heart failure. While rapidly advancing therapies preclude a definitive comprehensive guide, our goal is to present an up-to-date collection of topics that could serve as a useful adjunct to the classical textbooks. Particular emphasis is given to niche topics that are sometimes ignored in other works or are not as "glamorous" or high profile as topics such as transplantation and ventricular assist devices (all of which are worthy of entire texts themselves).

Most importantly, we, the editors, would like to thank all the authors for their tireless efforts on this project, which clearly represent an objective manifestation of their commitment to one of the most challenging areas of clinical medicine. The tremendous advances in the outcomes and improved survival of patients with heart failure are a testament to their dedication.

Giuseppe Rescigno
Department of Cardiothoracic Surgery
New Cross Hospital
Royal Wolverhampton Trust
Wolverhampton, United Kingdom

Michael S. Firstenberg, MD FACC
Chair, Cardiothoracic and Cardiovascular Surgery
The Medical Center of Aurora
Aurora, Colorado

Chair, The American College of Cardiology
Credentialing and Member Services Committee

Adjunct Faculty, College of Graduate Studies and
Associate Professor of Surgery and Integrative Medicine
Northeast Ohio Medical University
Rootstown, Ohio

Chapter 1

Introductory Chapter: Heart Failure - A Multifaceted Syndrome

Giuseppe Rescigno

Additional information is available at the end of the chapter

http://dx.doi.org/10.5772/intechopen.85478

1. Introduction

Heart failure (HF) is a worldwide issue. This syndrome is estimated to be present in more than 37 million of patients in the world [1]. In Western countries, this is mainly related to ischemic heart disease, hypertension and diabetes mellitus. In developing and Third-World countries, the causes are more varied. There is still a high incidence of rheumatic disease and end-stage valvulopathies. However, ischemic heart disease is increasing due to the spread of risk factors (diabetes, hypercholesterolemia, smoke). Progressive ageing of the population is another factor that has greatly increased the incidence of HF over the years. The number of hospital admissions with HF as a diagnosis in the USA tripled from 1.27 million in 1979 to 3.86 million in 2004 [2].

Nevertheless, despite major improvements of medical, interventional and surgical treatment, the mortality of the patients with advanced HF is still high; a recent analysis of Medicare patients showed a 50% mortality at 3 years [3].

Apart from the clinical burden in terms of morbidity and mortality, the financial impact of HF is impressive. A forecasting of the impact of heart failure in the USA showed an increase of total expenditure from 21 billion to 53 billion between 2012 and 2030 [4].

2. Classifications

The American College of Cardiology and AHA practice guidelines for chronic HF published in 2001 proposed a classification that includes four stages of HF [5]. Stages A and B are early phases without an overt syndrome and are alerting states. Stage A patients are at risk for HF related to conditions such as hypertension, atherosclerotic heart disease and diabetes mellitus. Stage B patients have developed structural heart disease from a variety of potential insults to the heart muscle, i.e. myocardial infarctions or valvular heart diseases, but still asymptomatic. Stages C and D are the symptomatic phases of HF. Therapeutic interventions, including dietary salt restriction, medications and implantable devices (pacemakers and defibrillators), are indicated for patients with symptomatic heart failure (stage C). In the end stages of HF (stage D), patients present marked symptoms at rest or with minimal activity despite optimal medical therapy.

Another important classification of HF is based on the left ventricular ejection fraction (EF) value. We generally consider the HF as a low (reduced, <40%) EF syndrome (HFrEF). There is indeed an almost equal number of patients in HF with a preserved EF (>50%) (HFpEF). In between we find patients with moderately reduced EF (40–49%, HFmrEF). The HFpEF shows normally a diastolic LV dysfunction [6].

3. Diagnosis

The diagnosis of HF may be sometimes challenging. There are the classical signs and symptoms that represent the definition of the syndrome (shortness of breath, fatigue, elevated JVP, crackles, ankle swelling, gallop rhythm). However, there are also less specific ones; for instance, depression could be a symptom of HF, as well as confusion, in particular in the elderly. In the older people, in particular, there may be other conditions that make the diagnosis more difficult (i.e. chronic pulmonary diseases). In stable patients, the measurements of natriuretic peptides may help. NT-proBNP level > 125 pg/mL or BNP level > 35 pg/mL should prompt the request for an echocardiography if one of the classical signs or symptoms is present [7]. Transthoracic echocardiography represents the cheapest assessment that may give a certain diagnosis. Care should be taken when an HFpEF is present. In these patients a diastolic, dysfunction should be demonstrated to make diagnosis.

Other imaging modalities could be used in doubtful cases as magnetic resonance imaging (MRI) or gated single-photon emission CT (SPECT). MRI is extremely accurate in measuring volumes, masses and EF of both ventricles. The gadolinium-enhanced modality allows a precise assessment of fibrosis, scars and inflammation (myocarditis). Amyloidosis, sarcoidosis, Chagas disease, non-compaction cardiomyopathy and haemochromatosis are similarly well defined by MRI [8].

4. Prevention

The value of prevention in HF has is now well established. The most effective way is a thorough control of hypertension if present [9]. A mild alcohol intake and a regular physical activity are also extremely beneficial. A prompt pharmacological intervention in asymptomatic patients is also recommended; the use of ACE inhibitors has clearly shown to reduce mortality and hospital admissions in patients without a clinically evident HF but with a low EF [10].

5. Treatment

The pharmacological treatment of HF is clearly codified in several national and international guidelines [11]. The cornerstones remain the diuretics, beta blockers, ACE inhibitors and mineralocorticoid receptor antagonists; recently new medications have been used with promising results in subcategories of HF patients like the ivabradine and sacubitril valsartan. However, a multidisciplinary discussion about every single patient and a close monitoring of the clinical effectiveness are important [12]. The management of acute HF decompensation is more complex and less codified.

HF patients may benefit of a few non-pharmacological interventions able mainly to improve survival. The mortality in HF is to be cancelled not infrequently sudden and related to arrhythmic events. The most recent guidelines about HF clearly states that 'An implantable cardioverter-defibrillator (ICD) is recommended to reduce the risk of sudden death and all-cause mortality in patients who have recovered from a ventricular arrhythmia causing haemodynamic instability, and who are expected to survive for >1 year with good functional status'. This is a recommendation IA, therefore with a very strong evidence. Moreover, the ICD is also strongly recommended in patients with an EF <35% after 3 months of optimal medical treatment and when life expectancy is more than 1 year [7]. On the contrary, when the patient is in NYHA Class IV and is not a candidate for cardiac resynchronisation therapy (CRT), ventricular assist device (VAD) or heart transplantation, the ICD is formally contraindicated.

The cardiac resynchronisation therapy (CRT) is a non-pharmacological/non-surgical treatment that represents a consistent adjunct for HF management. It consists in a synchronous pacing of both ventricles. There are clear indications, mainly related to ECG parameters and the clinical status of the patient [7]. Nowadays, the CRT devices have frequently defibrillating or pacing features. This treatment has shown to improve the quality of life and, partly, the survival of HF patients [13, 14]. However, there are non-responders to CRT that sometimes are difficult to identify before the implantation. As a rule, ischemic patients respond less favourably; on the contrary, female subjects are better responders.

The last resource for end-stage HF patients or when a refractory acute HF develops are mechanical circulatory support devices. In case of acute decompensation, extracorporeal, non-durable life support systems can be used to unload the ventricles. When the condition is chronic, a left ventricular assist device (LVAD) can be indicated. There are five conditions [15] that may prompt the consideration of a MCS:

A. Bridge to decision or bridge to bridge: The use of short-term MCS (ECMO) in patients with cardiogenic shock until haemodynamics and end-organ perfusion are stabilised, contraindications for long-term MCS are excluded (brain damage after resuscitation) and additional therapeutic options including long-term VAD therapy or heart transplant can be evaluated.

B. Bridge to candidacy: The use of MCS (usually LVAD) to improve end-organ function in order to make an ineligible patient eligible for heart transplantation.

C. Bridge to transplantation: The use of MCS (LVAD or BiVAD) to keep the patient alive who is otherwise at high risk of death before transplantation until a donor organ becomes available.

D. Bridge to recovery: The use of MCS (typically LVAD) to keep the patient alive until the heart recovers enough to remove MCS.

E. Destination therapy: The long-term use of MCS (LVAD) as an alternative to transplantation in patients with end-stage HF ineligible for transplantation or long-term waiting for heart transplantation.

The technology behind LVAD is continuously evolving, and smaller and less invasive models are expected in the next few years.

Heart transplantation still represents a viable treatment modality for end-stage heart failure. Major issues are the shortage of donor organs and many possible complications like organ rejection, neoplasms, coronary artery disease of the graft, infections and renal failure. The indications and contraindications are well codified [16]. There is no randomised study; however, survival and quality of life are greatly improved. Management of immunosuppressant medications is of outmost importance.

6. Conclusion

Heart failure is a worldwide health issue; however, new diagnostic modalities, drugs, devices and multidisciplinary approaches will certainly be able to better manage these complex patients.

Author details

Giuseppe Rescigno

Address all correspondence to: grescigno@mac.com

Department of Cardiothoracic Surgery, New Cross Hospital, Royal Wolverhampton Trust, Wolverhampton, United Kingdom

References

[1] Bui AL, Horwich TB, Fonarow GC. Epidemiology and risk profile of heart failure. Nature Reviews. Cardiology. 2011;**8**:30-41

[2] Fang J, Mensah GA, Croft JB, Keenan NL. Heart failure-related hospitalization in the U. S., 1979 to 2004. Journal of the American College of Cardiology. 2008;**52**:428-434

[3] Chen J, Normand SL, Wang Y, Krumholz HM. National and regional trends in heart failure hospitalization and mortality rates for medicare beneficiaries, 1998–2008. Journal of the American Medical Association. 2011;**306**:1669-1678

[4] Heidenreich PA, Albert NM, Allen LA, Bluemke DA, Butler J, Fonarow GC, et al. Forecasting the impact of heart failure in the United States: A policy statement from the American Heart Association. Circulation. Heart Failure. 2013;**6**:606-619

[5] Hunt SA, Baker DW, Chin MH, Cinquegrani MP, Feldman AM, Francis GS, et al. ACC/AHA guidelines for the evaluation and management of chronic heart failure in the adult: Executive summary: A report of the American College of Cardiology/American Heart Association Task Force on Practice Guidelines (Committee to Revise the 1995 Guidelines for the Evaluation and Management of Heart Failure). Circulation. 2001;**104**:2996-3007

[6] McMurray JJV, Adamopoulos S, Anker SD, et al. ESC guidelines for the diagnosis and treatment of acute and chronic heart failure 2012: The task force for the diagnosis and treatment of acute and chronic heart failure 2012 of the European Society of Cardiology. Developed in collaboration with the heart. European Journal of Heart Failure. 2012;**14**: 803-869

[7] Ponikowski P, Voors AA, Anker SD, et al. ESC guidelines for the diagnosis and treatment of acute and chronic heart failure: The task force for the diagnosis and treatment of acute and chronic heart failure of the European Society of Cardiology (ESC) developed with the special contribution of the heart failure association (HFA) of the ESC. European Heart Journal. 2016;**37**:2129-2200

[8] Gonzalez JA, Kramer CM. Role of imaging techniques for diagnosis, prognosis and management of heart failure patients: Cardiac magnetic resonance. Current Heart Failure Reports. 2015;**12**:276-283

[9] Wright JT, Williamson JD, Whelton PK, et al. A randomized trial of intensive versus standard blood-pressure control. The New England Journal of Medicine. 2015;**373**:2103-2116

[10] The SOLVD Investigators. Effect of enalapril on mortality and the development of heart failure in asymptomatic patients with reduced left ventricular ejection fractions. The New England Journal of Medicine. 1992;**327**:685-691

[11] Available from: https://www.nice.org.uk/guidance/ng106/chapter/Putting-this-guideline-into-practice

[12] McMurray JJ, Packer M, Desai AS, Gong J, Lefkowitz MP, Rizkala AR, et al. PARADIGM-HF Investigators and committees. Angiotensin-neprilysin inhibition versus enalapril in heart failure. The New England Journal of Medicine. 2014;**371**:993-1004

[13] Cleland JG, Abraham WT, Linde C, et al. An individual patient meta-analysis of five randomized trials assessing the effects of cardiac resynchronization therapy on morbidity and mortality in patients with symptomatic heart failure. The European Heart Journal. 2013;**34**:3547-3556

[14] Sohaib SMMA, Finegold JA, Nijjer SS, et al. Opportunity to increase life span in narrow QRS cardiac resynchronization therapy recipients by deactivating ventricular pacing: Evidence from randomized controlled trials. JACC Heart Fail. 2015;**3**:327-336

[15] Stewart GC, Givertz MM. Mechanical circulatory support for advanced heart failure: Patients and technology in evolution. Circulation. 2012;**125**:1304-1315

[16] Mehra MR, Canter CE, Hannan MM, et al. The 2016 International Society for heart lung transplantation listing criteria for heart transplantation: A 10-year update. The Journal of Heart and Lung Transplantation. 2016;**35**:1-23

Chapter 2

Telemedicine for Chronic Heart Failure: An Update

Emmanuel Andrès, Samy Talha,
Mohamed Hajjam and Amir Hajjam El Hassani

Additional information is available at the end of the chapter

http://dx.doi.org/10.5772/intechopen.80251

Abstract

Background: This is a short narrative review of the literature pertaining to telemedicine projects developed in the field of chronic heart failure (CHF), with particular focus on non-invasive telemonitoring projects including the French ones.

Results: Numerous non-invasive telemonitoring projects based on connected objects and information and communication technology (ICT) have emerged in the CHF field over the last 10 years. Others are under development, such as the main international randomized telemonitoring studies TELE-HF, TIM-HF, and BEAT-HF, or the French telemonitoring projects SCAD, OSICAT, PIMS, MEDICA, and E-care. The E-care project is a new-generation project supporting patients' returning home after hospital discharge. It perfectly fits within the framework of telemedicine 2.0 projects, including for the first time artificial intelligence (AI). This project has been specifically designed to automatically detect situations at risk for CHF. The potential contribution of these French projects (OSICAT, E-care), in terms of mortality, morbidity, number of hospitalizations prevented, as well as economic benefits, is currently studied or documented.

Keywords: telemedicine, telemonitoring, artificial intelligence, information and communication technology, Web, Telemedicine 2.0, chronic heart failure, diabetes mellitus, chronic disease

1. Introduction

The rising prevalence of chronic diseases, such as chronic heart failure (CHF) or metabolic disorders, combined with population aging, represents a major public health problem [1]. A prevalence of over 5.8 million affected people has been reported in the USA, and of over 26 million people worldwide. In France, between 120,000 and 150,000 new cases of CHF are diagnosed every year [2]. The cost of this chronic disease has rocketed, and is currently estimated at several billion dollars in developed countries [1].

The management of CHF patients proves challenging for healthcare professionals, since CHF remains a serious disease in terms of functional prognosis, survival prognosis, and associated morbidity and mortality [1]. The mortality rate of CHF patients in Stage III–IV according to the New York Heart Association (NYHA) classification is 50% at 5 years (30% in more recent studies), approaching that of metastatic breast cancer [2, 3].

Moreover, CHF patients are frequently admitted for emergency hospitalization and re-hospitalization [1, 2]. In France, CHF is responsible for more than 100,000 hospitalizations per year [2], accounts for 5% of all hospitalizations, and is the first cause of hospitalization among elderly subjects [2]. Some of these hospitalizations could be prevented if patients had a better follow-up [1]. This last point has been particularly well documented in the field of CHF [1, 4].

CHF management requires extensive medical resources, just at a time when medical shortage is beginning to be felt, along with medical deserts and poor access to medical care, among other problems.

In this setting, telemedicine may be of real help. Indeed, heart failure (HF) telemedicine, particularly HF telemonitoring, may optimize the management of such chronic diseases, particularly by preventing emergency and repeated hospitalizations [2, 4].

In this article, we have reviewed the literature on telemedicine for CHF, with a particular focus on non-invasive HF telemonitoring and French HF telemedicine projects.

2. Search strategy

A literature search was performed on the *PubMed* database of the *US National Library of Medicine* and on *Google Scholar*. We searched for articles published between January 2010 and April 2018, using the following keywords or associations: "*chronic heart failure*", "*telemedicine*", "*telemonitoring*", "*telemedicine in chronic heart failure*", and "*telemonitoring in chronic heart failure*"; restrictions included: English- or French-language publications; published from January 1, 2010, to May 1, 2018; human subjects; clinical trials, review articles or guidelines.

Information and data collected from international meetings were also used, as was information from commercial sites on the *Web*.

All English and French abstracts were reviewed by at least two senior researchers from our working group on telemedicine in chronic diseases at the *University Hospital of Strasbourg* (Strasbourg, France), a referral center. After rigorous selection, only 30 papers were included in our review and analyzed. Only completed telemedicine projects meeting rigorous clinical evaluation, *e.g.*, using evidence-based medicine criteria or criteria usually used for clinical trials, were included in this work. Additional data retrieved from the *Web* (references [5–37]) were also used to enable us to write this chapter in the form of a narrative review. This review is limited by its focus on non-invasive CHF telemonitoring.

3. First-generation heart failure telemonitoring projects

Since the beginning of the 2000's, numerous telemedicine projects have been conceived and developed in the area of CHF [5–21]. Practically all of them investigated "*telemonitoring*" (or telemanagement, as also termed in the literature), as defined under French legislation [22]. It should be noted that several systematic reviews pertaining to this medical field have been published in recent years [4, 16]. Nevertheless, in our opinion, these papers do not provide a general idea of the studies carried out, given that they were mainly restricted to morbidity and mortality studies (**Table 1**). To the best of our knowledge, no completed projects on "*teleconsultation*" or "*tele-expertise*" in the CHF area have been published so far. These terms are defined in **Table 2**.

Some of the projects specifically investigated CHF in subjects aged over 75 or 80 years, yielding good results [6, 23]. They are of special interest in ("real-life") practice, given that the mean age of CHF patients in developed countries approximates 80 years.

It is worth bearing in mind that these projects, particularly the earlier ones, more closely resembled a telephone follow-up with care providers (such as a nurse) traveling to the patient's home ("*structured telephone monitoring*" (**Table 2**)), rather than telemedicine as we consider it nowadays, with nonintrusive, automated, smart telemonitoring using remote sensors and modern communication technology or even artificial intelligence (AI) ("*telemedicine 2.0*") (**Table 2**) [4, 20]. Hence, in our opinion, these studies represent the first generation of telemedicine projects [4, 14].

3.1. Clinical impact of first-generation non-invasive heart failure telemonitoring

As we will see, the results of telemedicine projects conducted so far in the CHF field differed from study to study, with fairly inconclusive results as to the potential clinical benefits in terms

Overall mortality	Therapeutic education
Heart failure mortality	Hygiene-dietary and therapeutic compliance
Hospitalization for heart failure	Optimization of food and sports hygiene
Re-hospitalization for heart failure	Patient self-management
Number of hospitalization days	
	Optimization of the care pathway
Health costs	Structuring of the care pathway
Heart failure management costs	
Number of days off work	City-hospital relations
	Information sharing among health professionals
Quality of life	System use by health professionals

Table 1. Potential parameters to be evaluated in a telemedicine project on heart failure.

Telemedicine	Provision of remote patient care and consultation using telecommunication technologies.
Telemonitoring (telesurveillance)	This telemedicine practice allows a healthcare professional to remotely interpret the data necessary for the patient's medical follow-up in order to make decisions about his / her care. Remote data collection from a patient through a connected device or questionnaires to monitor his/her vital parameters and symptoms at home on a daily basis.
Tele-expertise	This practice of telemedicine consists, for a medical professional, to seek the opinion of one or more medical professional experts regarding elements of the patient's medical file. Remote seeking by a health professional of a second medical opinion via sending of images (scanner, X-ray, eye fundus, etc.) and sometimes exchange by Internet-based videoconference.
Teleconsultation	This telemedicine practice allows a medical professional to hold a consultation with a patient remotely. In the context of a teleconsultation, the patient can have at his/her side a health professional assisting the remote professional as well as a psychologist. Second opinion consultation by specialist.
Structured telephone monitoring	This basic concept of care reaching beyond the health care setting relies on a simple phone call monitoring strategy where patient compliance, symptoms, vital signs, and weight are followed remotely.
Telemedicine 2.0	Over the last decade, the Internet has become increasingly popular and is now an important part of our daily life. The use of "Web 2.0" technologies in health/medicine care or in telemedicine is referred to as "Health 2.0" or "Medicine 2.0", and "telemedicine 2.0".
Artificial intelligence	This concept describes the simulation of human intelligence processes by machines, especially computer systems. These processes include learning (the acquisition of information and rules for using the information), reasoning (using the rules to reach approximate or definite conclusions) and self-correction. Particular applications of AI include expert systems, speech recognition, and machine vision.

Table 2. Glossary of terms and definitions in the field of telemedicine, as proposed by the Italian Association of Hospital Cardiologists, the Italian Society of Cardiology and the Italian Society for Telemedicine and eHealth on telemedicine and as laid out in article 36 of the French social security financing (adapted from w.ncbi.nlm.nih.gov [last accessed: April 2018] and references [1, 2]).

of re-hospitalization and decreased morbidity or mortality [5–21], particularly regarding the statistical significance of the results. As a consequence, experts have now widely divergent opinions on the actual utility of telemedicine in CHF patient management. Of note is that the European Society of Cardiology (ESC) has, nevertheless, recommended telemedicine with a low level of evidence for such patient follow-up [24].

The 2016 ESC Guidelines for the diagnosis and treatment of acute and chronic HF for the first time recommended *"remote patient monitoring"* of CHF patients with a Grade of recommendation IIb, level of evidence B [25]. In this setting, telemonitoring is mainly focused on predicting acute decompensation episodes that are usually associated with fluid congestion and require therapy optimization (uptitration of angiotensin-converting enzyme inhibitors and beta-blockers). Clinical practice guidelines on CHF recommend daily weight measurements and define weight increases of >2 Kg per day as a warning alert.

It should be pointed out that the first studies on telemedicine for CHF were at times conducted with inappropriate methodologies, involving unsuitable patient groups (such as NYHA Stage

http://dx.doi.org/10.5772/intechopen.80251

I) and small-sized patient samples (between 50 and 1000 patients), with very short follow-up periods (between 3 months and 1 year) [5–21]. Moreover, most of these studies were based only on weight variations, without including other warning or monitoring parameters (*see* **Table 2**). In our opinion, these drawbacks rendered any clinical benefits demonstrated illusory [4, 20].

The *Trans-European Network - Home-Care Management System* (TEN-HMS) study, conducted in 2005, was the first larger study that analyzed telemonitoring's role in selected HF patients [25]. In this study, 426 patients were randomly assigned to "*telemonitoring*", "*nurse telephone support*", or "*usual care*" in a 2:2:1 ratio. Telemonitoring allowed data transfer (weight, blood pressure, ECG) to a central Web server via a conventional telephone line, and then to workstations based at each investigator site via secure intranet connections. Patients were invited to proceed to data transfer twice daily. Values greater or lower than the predefined limits were signaled automatically to study nurses who could either provide directly advice to the patient or, in more severe cases, inform the primary care physician. In addition to usual care, patients in the group with nurse telephone support were allowed to contact the HF-specialist nurse by telephone at any time during office hours. Additionally, the nurse contacted the patients by telephone every month in order to assess their symptoms and current medication and provide advice. In comparison with usual care alone, mortality and re-hospitalization rates were proven lower in the groups receiving either telemonitoring or nurse telephone support, with no statistically significant differences between both latter intervention groups. Of note is that the hospital stay duration, and therefore the time until outpatient care was deemed sufficient, was 6 days less in the group of patients receiving telemonitoring.

Name of the study	Method	Results
Tele-HF study [17]	Telemonitoring (n = 826) *vs.* standard care (n = 827)	The study found no significant difference between the telemonitoring and standard management groups in terms of all-cause readmission or all-cause mortality in the 180 days following inclusion (odds ratio [OR]: 1.04 [95% CI: 0.91–1.19]) (p = ns). The primary endpoint, all-cause readmission or death within 180 days after enrollment, occurred in 52.3% of the telemonitoring group and 51.5% of the usual care group.
TIM-HF study [18]	Telemonitoring (n = 354) *vs.* standard care (n = 356)	The all-cause mortality rate was 8.4 per 100 patient-years of follow-up in the telemedicine group and 8.7 per 100 patient-years of follow-up in the standard care group (OR: 0.97 [95%CI: 0.67–1.41]; $p = 0.87$).
BEAT-HF Study [26]	Intervention group, which included pre-discharge HF education, regularly scheduled telephone coaching, and remote monitoring of weight, blood pressure, heart rate, and symptoms (n = 715), *vs.* usual care group (n = 722)	The rate of all-cause readmission at 180 days was 51% in the intervention group *vs.* 49% in the control group ($p = 0.74$). 30-day readmission rate: 23% *vs.* 22% (p = 0.63) for intervention *vs.* control group, respectively, and 30-day mortality: 3.4% *vs.* 5.4% ($p = 0.06$) for intervention *vs.* control group. 180-day mortality: 14% *vs.* 16% ($p = 0.34$) for intervention *vs.* control group respectively.

Table 3. Results of the main international randomized studies on telemonitoring in heart failure.

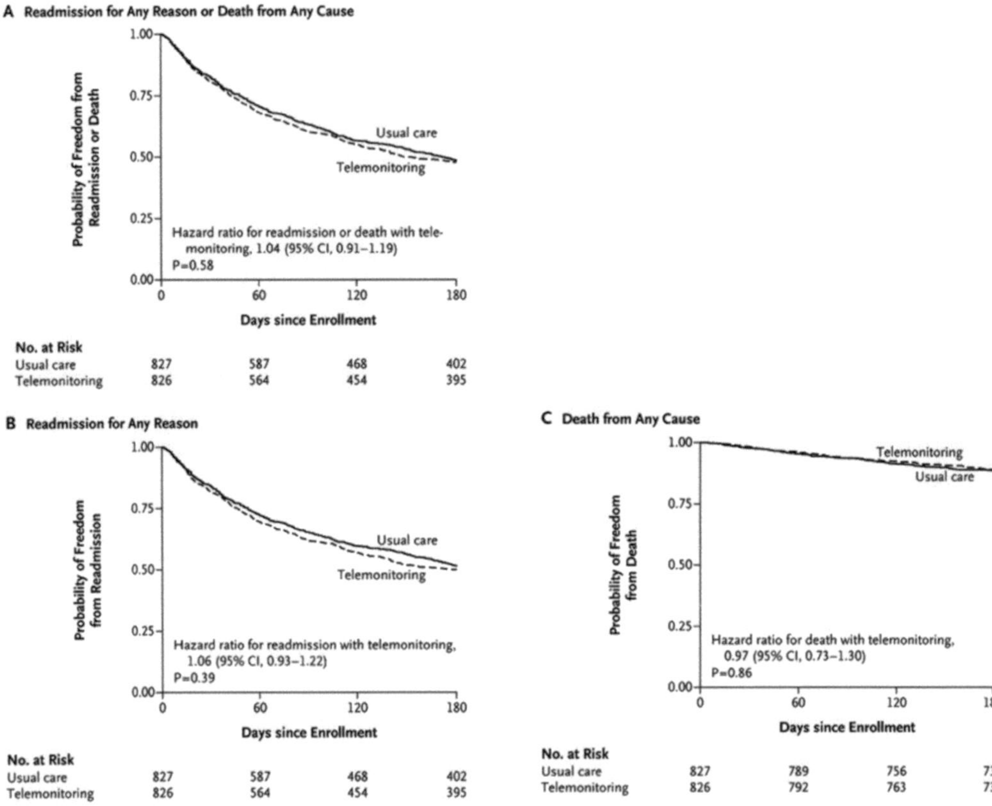

Figure 1. Tele-HF trial (n = 1653 patients included). Primary endpoint: "readmission for any reason" and "death from any cause", and each component separately, according to treatment group (n = 1653) (*adapted from* http://www.nejm.org/doi/full/10.1056/NEJMoa1010029 [last accessed: May 2018] and reference [17]).

Despite some limitations, several reviews and meta-analyses have apparently shown an undeniable utility of telemedicine [4, 16]. For instance, Inglis et al. [16] reported that telemedicine had an effect on all-cause mortality, which fell significantly by 34% ($p < 0.0001$) in the study they conducted. They also revealed a 20% decrease in the number re-hospitalizations for CHF, an improvement of the patient's quality of life and management costs, and a good acceptance of the system. In the meta-analysis by Anker et al. [4], 11 studies were analyzed as part of a comparison between the effects of telemonitoring (non-invasive telemedicine) and routine care. Their research revealed that telemonitoring led to a reduction in all-cause mortality (10.4% *vs*. 15.4%; $p < 0.0001$), all-cause hospitalization (47.2% *vs*. 52.1%; $p = 0.02$), and hospitalization for CHF (22.4% *vs*. 28.5%; $p = 0.008$).

Conversely, three prospective clinical trials, the "gold standard", displayed results contradicting the previous ones and thus questioned the potential utility of telemedicine in CHF [17, 18, 26] (**Table 3**). In the Tele-HF study, patients hospitalized for CHF were randomized to telemonitoring with voice-based interactive structured telephone support (n = 826) or standard care (n = 827) [17]. Patients in the intervention arm were asked to call a toll-free telephone system and answer a series of questions regarding their general health, weight, and HF symptoms on a daily basis. A clinician then analyzed this information. No significant difference was found between the telemonitoring and standard management groups in terms of all-cause readmission or all-cause mortality in the 180 days following inclusion (odds ratio [OR]: 1.04 [95% CI: 0.91–1.19]) (**Figure 1**). The primary outcome, all-cause readmission or death within 180 days after enrollment, occurred in 52.3% of the telemonitoring group patients and 51.5% of the usual care group. However, adherence was poor despite system-generated reminders, given that 14% of patients in the telemonitoring arm of the study never used the system. By the final week, only 55% of the patients were using the system at least three times a week.

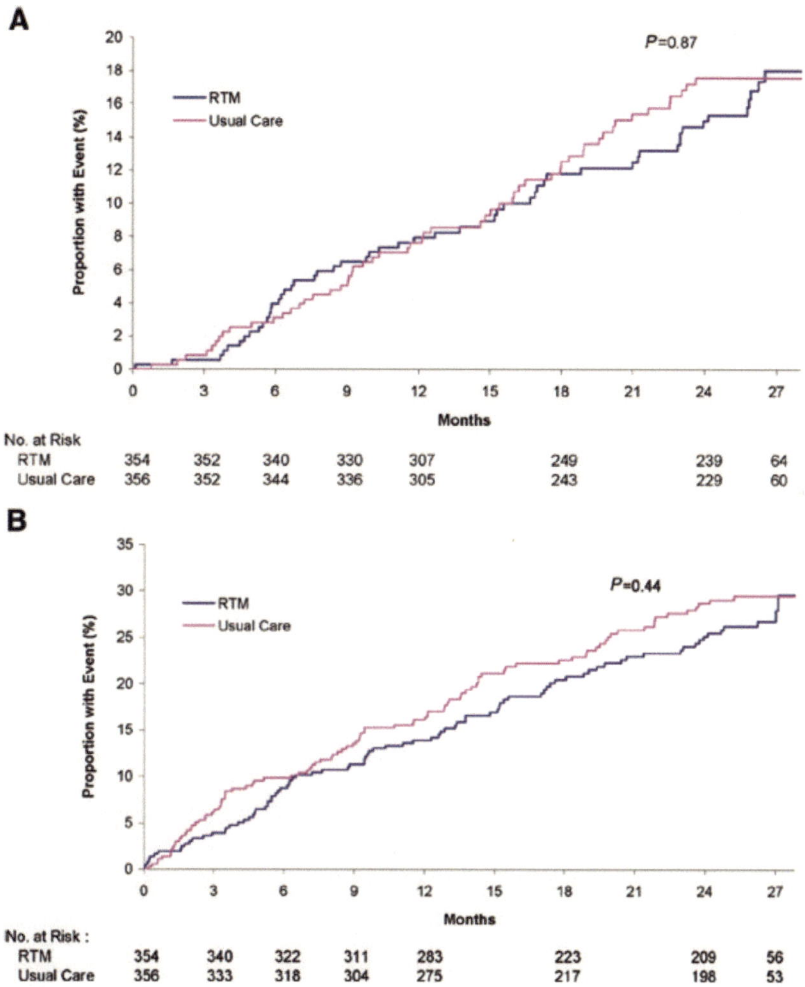

Figure 2. TIM-HF trial (n = 710). (a): Primary endpoint: "death from any cause"; and (B): Composite secondary endpoint: "Hospitalization for heart failure" or "cardiovascular death" during follow-up. RTM refers to remote telemedical management (*adapted from* http://circ.ahajournals.org/content/circulationaha/123/17/1873.full.pdf [last accessed: May 2018] and reference [17]).

The TIM-HF study, conducted in Germany, involved 710 stable CHF patients who were randomly assigned to one of the following two groups: 1) telemonitoring by means of remote monitoring and telephone support (n = 354); standard care (n = 356) [18]. Patients were given a personal digital assistant (PDA) with a wireless *Bluetooth* interface. The system collected ECG data, blood pressure readings, and body weight, which were then communicated wirelessly to a central location where a physician was present 24 hours a day, 7 days a week. In this study, the all-cause mortality rate was 8.4 per 100 patient-years of follow-up in the telemedicine group and 8.7 per 100 patient-years of follow-up in the standard care group (OR: 0.97 [95% CI: 0.67–1.41]; $p = 0.87$) (**Figure 2**). The TIM-HF trial was, however, underpowered to detect a significant difference in mortality between the two groups. The composite secondary outcome of hospitalization for HF and death due to a cardiovascular cause (14.7% *vs*. 16.5%) highlighted the stable nature of HF patients recruited into the study as compared to the population- and trial-based readmission rates approaching 50% reported in the literature.

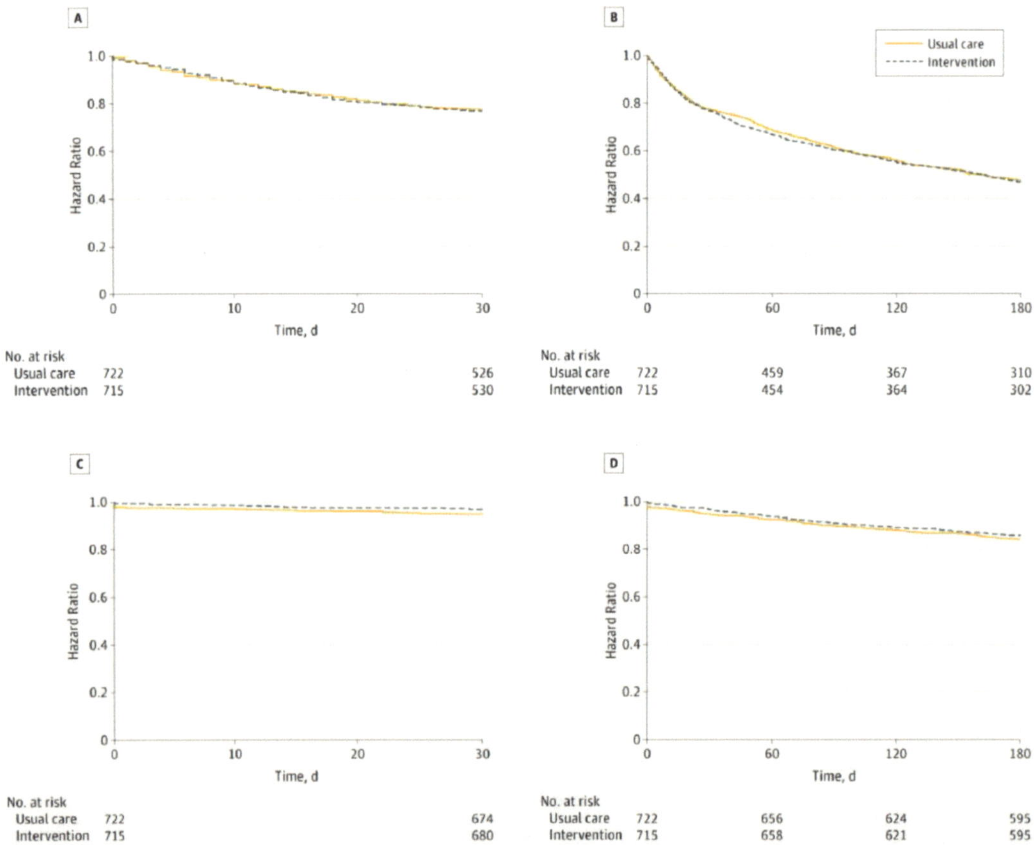

Figure 3. BEAT-HF trial (n = 1437). (A): 30-day readmission; (B): 180-day readmission; (C): 30-day mortality with the intervention; and (D): 180-day mortality (adapted from https://www.ncbi.nlm.nih.gov/pmc/articles/PMC4827701/ [last accessed: May 2018] and reference [26]).

Thereafter, only one large study on remote monitoring of this kind has been published, namely the BEAT-HF trial, which produced negative results, despite the inclusion of 1437 patients after cardiac decompensation [26]. In this study, there was no significant difference between the "intervention" group, involving pre-discharge HF education, regularly scheduled telephone coaching, and remote monitoring of weight, blood pressure, heart rate, and symptoms, and the "usual care" group regarding all-cause readmissions 180 days after discharge, which occurred in 50.8% (363 of 715) and 49.2% (355 of 722) of patients, respectively (adjusted hazard ratio: 1.03 [95% CI: 0.88–1.20]; $p = 0.74$) (**Figure 3**). In secondary analyses, while 30-day readmission or 180-day mortality did not significantly differ between both groups, there was a significant difference in 180-day quality of life between the intervention and usual care groups. No adverse events were reported.

3.2. Financial impact of first-generation non-invasive heart failure telemonitoring

Aside from these medical considerations, it is worth noting that all the studies seem to agree that using telemedicine solutions in CHF management proved at least economically beneficial (**Table 1**) [5–20]. Depending on the study, the savings were estimated at between $5000 and >$50,000/year/patient according to the CHF stage and study setting. In the study by Scalvini et al. [21], the cost of CHF patient management fell by 24%, and hospital costs fell by €45,186/patient/year.

In this context, the study by Burdese et al. [6] proves to be one of the most convincing for illustrating the utility of telemanagement in CHF elderly patients. In this study, a significant reduction was observed in re-hospitalizations (35 without *vs.* 12 with telemedicine, $p = 0.0001$), emergency department visits for an acute HF episode (21 *vs.* 5/year, $p = 0.0001$), and management costs (€116,856 *vs.* €40,065/year). Interestingly, only 8.6% of patients discontinued telemanagement, demonstrating that it was well accepted.

4. Ongoing French heart failure telemedicine projects

4.1. General data

Over the last 4 to 5 years, a second generation of projects has emerged in the CHF area, particularly in France [20, 27–32]. These projects are known as *"telemedicine 2.0"*, because they utilize the new information and communication technology (ICT) and the Internet. They meet the requirements of telemedicine, as laid out in Article 36 of the French Social Security Financing Act (**Table 1**) [22].

Most of these projects use the common connected tools for CHF monitoring (*"multi-channels"* or *"multi-sensors"*), such as blood pressure meters, weighing scales, and pulse oximeters, which transmit the collected information via *Bluetooth, 3G,* or *4G,* along with tools for interaction between the patient and healthcare professionals, such as telephone support centers, tablets, and websites [20]. Some projects also include tools for motivation and education, and occasionally, questionnaires about symptoms, such as *"dyspnea"*, *"palpitation"* and *"edema"*, as experienced by the patient. Most of these studies also include AI tools.

4.2. Main non-invasive heart failure telemonitoring projects in France

The main telemedicine projects that are currently being developed in France are:

- SCAD: *"Suivi CArdiologique à Distance"* [remote cardiological follow-up], first initiated in 2005, deployed in Lower Normandy, France, between 2009 April and May 2012, and developed by the Caen University Hospital (Caen, France) [27];
- PIMPS: *"Plateforme Interactive Médecins Patients Santé"* [doctor–patient interactive health platform], initiated in 2013, developed by the René-Dubos hospital in Pontoise (Pontoise, France) [28];
- OSICAT: *"Optimisation de la Surveillance ambulatoire des Insuffisants CArdiaques par Télécardiologie"* [optimization of outpatient monitoring in heart failure patients using telecardiology], initiated in 2012 and involving 12 local investigation centers coordinated by the Toulouse University Hospital (Toulouse, France) [29];
- MEDICA: *"Monitorage Electronique à Domicile de l'Insuffisance CArdiaque chronique"* [electronic home-monitoring of chronic heart failure], initiated in 2014 and developed by the REUNICA domicile and GMC-solutions santé groups working in the social protection of the elderly [30];
- E-care: *"Détection des situations à risque de décompensation cardiaque chez les patients insuffisants cardiaques de stade III de la NYHA"* [detection of risk situations for cardiac decompensation in heart failure patients with NYHA Stage-III disease], initiated in 2014, with the project's medical aspects developed by the Strasbourg University Hospital (Strasbourg, France) [31, 32].

All these projects make use of the telemedicine 2.0 tools discussed above. The PIMPS project also comprises laboratory monitoring of natriuretic peptide [26]. The projects focus on CHF patient cohorts or prospective studies. They have enrolled relatively large patient samples, and most of them are based on data derived from evidence-based medicine. The OSICAT study, which seems the most advanced [29], was launched in 2013 and has enrolled 990 patients divided into two groups: remote home monitoring (intervention group) and standard care (control group). The results, which are expected by 2018, will comprise an assessment of medical efficacy and cost-effectiveness.

The E-care telemonitoring project, conducted in Strasbourg, falls under this *"telemedicine 2.0"* category [31, 32]. It has been developed to optimize home monitoring of CHF patients by detecting, via a telemonitoring 2.0 platform, situations in which there is a risk of cardiac decompensation and re-hospitalization. The E-care platform automatically generates indicators of *"health status"* deterioration, *i.e.*, *"warning alerts"* for any chronic disease worsening, particularly CHF, that may lead to hospitalization if not treated. To our knowledge, it is the first project that uses AI in addition to ICT. The platform comprises connected nonintrusive medical sensors, a touchscreen tablet connected by *Wi-Fi,* and a router or *3G/4G,* making it possible to interact with the patient and provide education on treatment, diet, and lifestyle (**Figure 4**). The E-care system involves a server that hosts the patient's data and a secure *internet* portal to which the patient and hospital- and non-hospital-based healthcare professionals can connect. E-care is based on a smart system comprising an inference engine and a medical ontology for personalized synchronous or asynchronous analysis of data specific to each patient and, if necessary, the sending of an AI-generated alert [33].

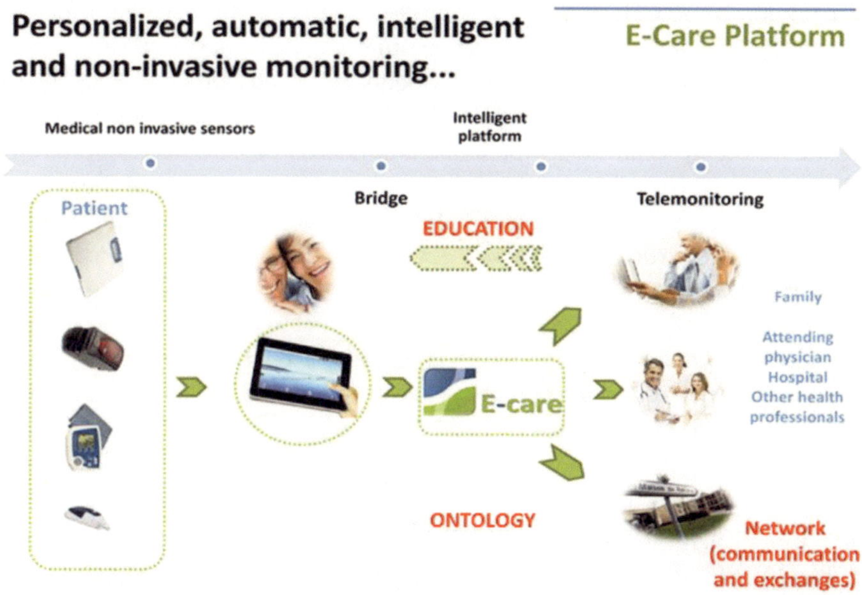

Figure 4. Version 1 of the generic telemedicine platform developed as part of the E-care telemonitoring project in heart failure patients. This platform utilized nonintrusive medical sensors measuring blood pressure, heart rate, oxygen saturation, and weight connected by Bluetooth and relaying real-time physiological data on the health status of the patient; touchscreen tablets connected by Wi-Fi or 3G/4G; Internet server hosting an inference engine that generated the warning alerts. These alerts indicated a deterioration in the patient's chronic diseases, especially chronic heart failure. Health professionals could access them via a secure Internet portal (adapted from [last accessed: May 2018] and reference [31]).

4.3. Clinical impact of the French non-invasive heart failure telemonitoring projects

To date, clinical results are only available for the SCAD and E-care projects [27, 32, 34]. In the SCAD project, 90 patients were randomized between April 2009 and May 2011 (n = 45 for each group) (thesis from the Faculty of Medicine of Caen, France, and reference [27]). The population was composed of elderly patients (mean age of 78 ± 6 years), mostly of male gender (78%), and at high risk of re-hospitalization (mean brain natriuretic peptide [BNP] level of 1025 ± 950 pg./mL). At 12 months, 1040 days of hospitalization for acute HF were recorded. Monitoring by educational telemedicine significantly reduced the number of hospital days for acute HF: 590 days in the control group *vs.* 450 days in the telemedicine group ($p = 0.044$). The endpoint *"death or hospitalization for acute heart failure"* occurred less frequently in the telemedicine group: 57.8% in the *control group vs.* 35.6% in the *telemedicine group* ($p < 0.05$). In case of CHF-related readmissions, telemedicine-treated patients had lower intra-hospital mortality: 18.2% *vs.* 0% ($p < 0.02$).

Between February 2014 and April 2015, 175 patients were given the opportunity to participate in the E-care project [31]. During this period, patients and healthcare professionals had to use the E-care platform on a daily basis according to a predefined protocol specific to each patient. The patients' mean age was 72 years, and the male-to-female ratio was 0.7. The patients had multiple comorbidities, with a mean Charlson comorbidity index of 4.1, the five more common being CHF in >60% of subjects, anemia in >40%, atrial fibrillation in 30%, type II diabetes in 30%, and chronic obstructive pulmonary disease in 30%. During the study, 1500 measurements were taken in these 175 patients, with 700 alerts generated by the E-care system in 68 patients [34]. Some 107 subjects (61.1%) had no alerts during follow-up. When analyzing the follow-up of these 107 patients, it appeared that they did not have any clinically significant event that might have led to hospitalization. Analysis of the warning alerts showed that the E-care platform automatically and non-intrusively detected any worsening of the patient's health, particularly with respect to CHF. Indeed, it was for the latter condition that the system yielded the best sensitivity, specificity, and positive and negative predictive values of 100%, 72%, 90%, and 100%, respectively. The E-care platform also showed its ability to detect a health status deterioration while taking into account the multiple diseases of the patients studied, with sensitivity, specificity, and positive and negative predictive values of 100%, 30%, 89%, and 100%, respectively.

5. Perspectives regarding new telemedicine projects in France

5.1. In the field of chronic heart disease

As mentioned above, the E-care platform appears capable of preventing hospitalization by detecting early any deterioration in the patient's health status and by alerting the care providers so that they can take appropriate measures [31, 32]. As other ongoing projects, the E-care platform is capable of structuring the patients' care pathways, a major theme in medicine for our governments and authorities (**Table 1**). It also provides a way for healthcare professionals to exchange with each other and facilitates access to medical resources.

With this in mind, an enhanced version of the E-care platform will be experimented for at-home monitoring of HF patients as part of a project called PRADO INCADO (**Figure 5**) [33]. The project is being run by a group bringing together the Strasbourg University Hospital, the Alsatian regional health agency, the Bas-Rhin branch of France's national health insurance, and the company PREDIMED Technology. This project will allow us to conduct an in-depth study so as to improve diagnosis by machine learning and detect abnormalities early.

This is in line with the research by Mortazavi et al. on the utility of AI in managing CHF patients, particularly regarding the possibility of predicting re-hospitalization for CHF [35].

5.2. In the field of diabetes mellitus

In addition to CHF, diabetes and metabolic disorders are other potential application fields of telemedicine that are intensively investigated in France. Innovative projects are being developed or deployed, such as the PLASIDIA platform that is run by the *European Center for the Study of Diabetes* in Strasbourg (France) [36]. It is in this setting that we developed an upgraded version of the E-care platform in order to follow diabetic patients as part of the DIABETe project. The new version of the E-care platform should be deployed in "complex diabetic"

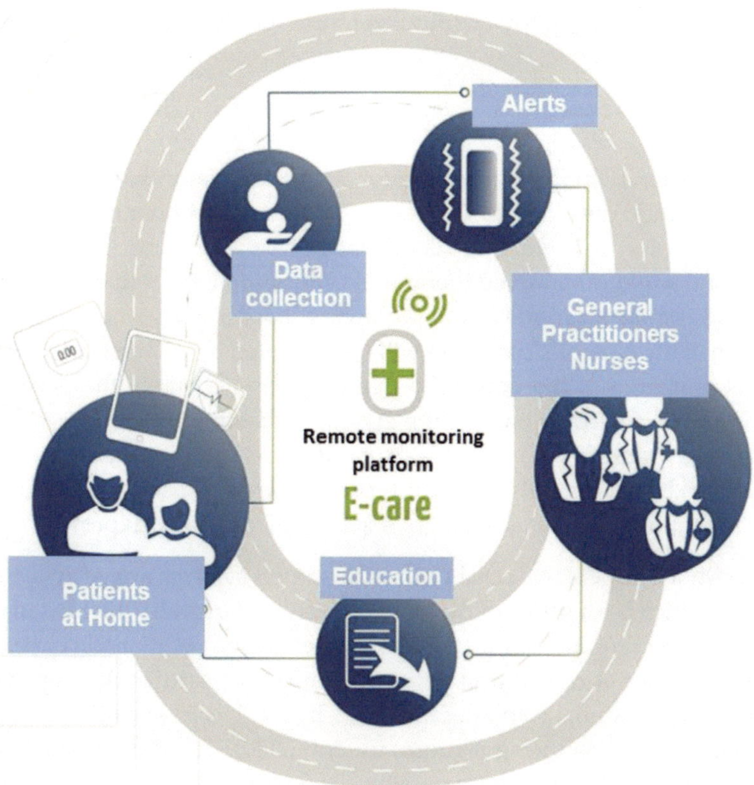

Figure 5. PRADO INCADO project. This project uses the E-care smart telemonitoring platform to follow heart failure patients at home according to the organizational model established by the national health insurance as part of the national PRADO program for heart failure patients, which aims to support heart failure patients returning home from hospital and to optimize their management. The PRADO INCADO project integrates a telemedicine solution to structure the patients' care pathways, enable healthcare professionals to exchange with each other, and incorporate a telemonitoring solution (*adapted from* https://www.omicsonline.org/open-access/telemedicine-to-monitor-elderly-patients-with-chronic-diseases-with-a-special-focus-on-patients-with-chronic-heart-failure-2167-7182-1000311.php?aid=73930 [last accessed: May 2018]).

patients, *e.g.*, diabetic patients at high cardiovascular risk or diabetic patients treated with multiple injections [37]. Most of these patients may develop an HF episode and possibly CHF over the long-term.

The DIABETe project is aimed at detecting early the risk of hospitalization in diabetic patients at "*very high cardiovascular risk*", defined as a personal history of myocardial infarction (MI) or stroke, limb amputation or cardiomyopathy, and "*intensive*" insulin therapy (at least 3 injections per day or pump), while offering them a personalized follow-up and education about their illness and its management [37]. This population is interesting, since it allows targeting polypathology and polymedication, and requires global support. It represents 50% of diabetics hospitalized in departments of diabetology and internal medicine.

Apart from cardiovascular complications (MI, arteritis obliterans of the lower limbs, etc.), these patients are also frequently hospitalized for hypoglycemia, diabetes imbalance, infections, etc.

The DIABETe project is based on an intelligent platform that will assist healthcare professionals by automatically processing the information obtained from nonintrusive medical sensors (blood glucose meter, blood pressure monitor, actimeter, connected scale, etc.) as well as the subjective information provided by the patient himself (questionnaires) and his/her behavior (compliance) in order to detect and report early these situations at risk of hospitalization [37]. Patient- and situation-adapted therapeutic education tools will be made available to the individual, and communication with the subject will occur via a touch pad. Alerts indicating a deterioration of the patient's condition will be generated by AI and transmitted to the health professionals in charge of the patient so that they can anticipate the decompensation and initiate appropriate measures outside the emergency setting. These innovative and original solutions derived from new technologies should achieve the best acceptability to patients. Medical data can be shared between health professionals as part of a city-hospital network. Ultimately, an improvement in the patient's quality of life is also expected.

DIABETe does not compete with Diabeo or other expert systems aimed at optimizing the glycemic balance, which is *per se* one of the main objectives of diabetes mellitus management [38]. The DIABETe project focuses on the "global" management of diabetic patients through the detection of situations at risk of hospitalization: infection, cardiac decompensation, diabetic foot, etc. but also of course hypoglycemia and hyperglycemia leading to hospitalizations. Regarding the remote monitoring platform used in DIABETe, an integration of or interfacing with expert systems such as Diabeo is possible. As a reminder, the Diabeo application, carried by Sanofi, was tested as part of the Télésage clinical trial in 700 patients with type 1 and type 2 diabetes treated with basal-bolus regimen (multiple injections or pump) [38]. The primary endpoint of the Télésage study was the HbA1c variation (glycemic control) at 1 year. A previous study, Télédiab1, conducted between 2007.

6. Conclusions

Though many non-invasive telemonitoring projects have been conducted in the CHF area, relatively few have been run in the setting of telemedicine 2.0 using ICT and the internet. The E-care telemonitoring project totally falls under this category. The potential utility of these projects in terms of morbidity, mortality, and hospitalization prevention is being studied or documented, and their health saving potential is also being investigated.

The telemedicine 2.0 projects are perfectly compatible with the care pathways that are being developed for chronic diseases by the French health authorities (including the French ministry of health and the regional branch of the national health insurance). What's more, all these findings should be analyzed with regard to the benefits provided by these telemedicine solutions (**Table 1**).

These fascinating developments will help shaping the medicine of tomorrow. In the field of chronic diseases, given the epidemiological situation and expected shortage of time careers, we need a better follow-up and better education of patients, an improved prevention and anticipation, and above all a better selection of healthcare system-dependent patients.

Declarations

Competing interests: Mohamed Hajjam is the scientific director of PREDIMED Technology.

Funding: Grant from the *Agence Régionale de Santé du Grand-Est*. Grant from the *Fondation de l'Avenir. Grant from the Agence Nationale de la Recherche (ANR) Technologie.*

Ethical approval: Not applicable.

Guarantor: Emmanuel Andrès.

Contributorship: Emmanuel Andrès and Samy Talha designed the study and conducted the literature searches. Emmanuel Andrès, Samy Talha, and Amir Hajjam El Hassani drafted the results and parts of the discussion. Samy Talha, Mohamed Hajjam, and Amir Hajjam El Hassani provided critical analysis, revised the whole manuscript, and approved the final version for publication. Emmanuel Andrès is responsible for all revisions and remains in contact with the rest of the review team regarding status reports.

Author details

Emmanuel Andrès[1,2*], Samy Talha[2,3], Mohamed Hajjam[4] and Amir Hajjam El Hassani[5]

*Address all correspondence to: emmanuel.andres@chru-strasbourg.fr

1 Department of Internal Medicine, Diabetes and Metabolic Diseases, Medical Clinic B, Strasbourg University Hospitals (Hôpitaux Universitaires de Strasbourg [HUS]), Strasbourg, France

2 Research Team EA 3072 "Mitochondria, Oxidative Stress and Muscle Protection", Faculty of Medicine of Strasbourg, University of Strasbourg (Université de Strasbourg [UdS]), Strasbourg, France

3 Department of Physiology and Functional Explorations, Strasbourg University Hospitals (Hôpitaux Universitaires de Strasbourg [HUS]), Strasbourg, France

4 PREDIMED Technology, Strasbourg, France

5 Research Team EA 4662 "Nanomedicine, Imaging, Therapeutics", University of Technology of Belfort-Montbéliard (Université de Technologie de Belfort-Montbéliard [UTBM]), Belfort-Montbéliard, France

References

[1] http://invs.santepubliquefrance.fr/publications/etat_sante_2017/ESP2017_Ouvrage_complet_vdef.pdf [April 2018]

[2] http://www.has-sante.fr/portail/upload/docs/application/pdf/2012-04/guide parcours de soins ic web.pdf [April 2018]

[3] Jessup M, Brozena S. Heart failure. The New England Journal of Medicine. 2003;**348**: 2007-2018

[4] Anker SD, Koehler F, Abraham WT. Telemedicine and remote management of patients with heart failure. Lancet. 2011;**378**:731-739

[5] Rosen D, McCall JD, Primack BA. Telehealth protocol to prevent readmission among high-risk patients with congestive heart failure. The American Journal of Medicine. 2017;**130**:1326-1330

[6] Burdese E, Testa M, Raucci P, Ferreri C, Giovannini G, Lombardo E, et al. Usefulness of a telemedicine program in refractory older congestive heart failure patients. Diseases. 2018;**6**:10. DOI: 10.3390/diseases6010010

[7] Feltner C, Jones CD, Cené CW, Zheng ZJ, Sueta CA, Coker-Schwimmer EJ, et al. Transitional care interventions to prevent readmissions for persons with heart failure: A systematic review and meta-analysis. Annals of Internal Medicine. 2014;**160**:774-784

[8] Martínez-González NA, Berchtold P, Ullman K, Busato A, Egger M. Integrated care programmes for adults with chronic conditions: A meta-review. International Journal for Quality in Health Care. 2014;**26**:561-570

[9] Achelrod D. Policy expectations and reality of telemedicine: A critical analysis of health care outcomes, costs and acceptance for congestive heart failure. Journal of Telemedicine and Telecare. 2014;**20**:192-200

[10] Pandor A, Thokala P, Gomersall T, Baalbaki H, Stevens JW, Wang J, et al. Home telemonitoring or structured telephone support programmes after recent discharge in patients with heart failure: Systematic review and economic evaluation. Health Technology Assessment. 2013;**17**:1-207

[11] Kraai IH, Luttik ML, de Jong RM, Jaarsma T, Hillege HL. Heart failure patients monitored with telemedicine: Patient satisfaction, a review of the literature. Journal of Cardiac Failure. 2011;**17**:684-690

[12] Dendale P, De Keulenaer G, Troisfontaines P, Weytjens C, Mullens W, Elegeert I, et al. Effect of a telemonitoring-facilitated collaboration between general practitioner and heart failure clinic on mortality and rehospitalization rates in severe heart failure: The TEMA-HF 1 (TElemonitoring in the MAnagement of heart failure) study. European Journal of Heart Failure. 2012;**14**:333-340

[13] Di Lenarda A, Caloso G, Gulizia MM, Aspromonte N, Scalvini S, Mortara A, et al. The future of telemedicine for the management of heart failure patients: A consensus document of the Italian Association of Hospital Cardiologists (A.N.M.C.O), the Italian Society of Cardiology (S.I.C.) and the Italian Society for Telemedicine and eHealth (Digital S.I.T.). Health Information Research. 2015;**21**:223-229

[14] http://www.thecochranelibrary.com/userfiles/ccoch/file/Telemedicine/CD007228.pdf [May 2018]

[15] Willemse E, Adriaenssens J, Dilles T, Remmen R. Do telemonitoring projects of heart failure fit the chronic care model? International Journal of Integrated Care. 2014;**14**:e023

[16] Inglis SC, Clark RA, McAlister FA, Ball J, Lewinter C, Cullington D, Stewart S, et al. Structured telephone support or telemonitoring programmes. Cochrane Database of Systematic Reviews. 2010;**8**:CD007228

[17] Chaudhry SI, Mattera JA, Curtis JP, Spertus JA, Herrin J, Lin Z, Phillips CO, et al. Telemonitoring in patients with heart failure. The New England Journal of Medicine. 2010;**363**:2301-2309

[18] Koehler F, Winkler S, Schieber M, Sechtem U, Stangl K, Böhm M, Boll H, et al. Impact of remote telemedical management on mortality and hospitalizations in ambulatory patients with chronic heart failure: The telemedical interventional monitoring in heart failure study. Circulation. 2011;**123**:1873-1880

[19] Kitsiou S, Paré G, Jaana M. Systematic reviews and meta-analyses of home telemonitoring interventions for patients with chronic diseases: A critical assessment of their methodological quality. Journal of Medical Internet Research. 2013;**15**:e150

[20] Andrès E, Talha S, Hajjam M, Hajjam J, Ervé S, Hajjam A. E-care project: A promising e-plateform for the optimizing management of chronic heart failure and other chronic diseases. Heart Research Open Journal. 2015;**1**:39-45

[21] Scalvini S, Capomolla S, Zanelli E, Benigno M, Domenighini D, Paletta L, et al. Effect of home-based telecardiology on chronic heart failure: Costs and outcomes. Journal of Telemedicine and Telecare. 2005;**11**(Suppl 1):16-18

[22] https://www.legifrance.gouv.fr/eli/arrete/2017/4/25/AFSH1711560A/jo/texte/fr [April 2018]

[23] Kaladjurdjevic M, Antonicelli R. Evaluation of motivation and attitude for Telehomecare among caregivers of elderly patients affected with congestive heart failure. Digital Medicine. 2016;**2**:149-156

[24] https://www.nvvc.nl/media/richtlijn/146/2016_Heartfailure.eurheartj.ehw128.full.pdf [May 2018]

[25] Cleland JGF. The trans-European network—Home-care management system (TEN-HMS) study: An investigation of the effect of telemedicine on outcomes in Europe. Disease Management and Health Outcomes. 2006;**14**(Suppl 1):23-28

[26] Ong MK, Romano PS, Edgington S, Aronow HU, Auerbach AD, Black JT, et al. Effectiveness of remote patient monitoring after discharge of hospitalized patients with heart FailureThe better effectiveness after transition–heart failure (BEAT-HF) randomized clinical trial. JAMA Internal Medicine. 2016;**176**:310-318

[27] http://www.telesante-basse-normandie.fr/l-enrs-et-les-projets/scad,1642,1346.html [April 2018]

[28] http://www.pimps.fr/[April 2018]

[29] http://www.osicat.fr/[April 2018]

[30] http://www.groupe.reunica.com/files/live/sites/reucorp/files/Vous Informer/Espace Presse/Dossiers/Dossierdepresse Reunica Domicile Dispositif de télémédecine a domicile pour insuffisance cardiaque chronique.pdf [April 2018]

[31] Andrès E, Talha S, Ahmed Benyahia A, Keller O, Hajjam M, Moukadem A, et al. Expérimentation d'une plateforme de détection automatisée des situations à risque de décompensation cardiaque (plateforme E-care) dans une unité de Médecine Interne. La Revue de Médecine Interne. 2016;**37**:587-593

[32] Andrès E, Talha S, Benyahia AA, Keller O, Hajjam M, Moukadem A, et al. E-health: A promising solution for the optimized management of chronic diseases. Example of a national e-health project E-care based on a e-plateform in the context of chronic heart failure. European Research in Telemedicine/La Recherche Européenne en Télémédecine. 2015;**4**:87-94

[33] Ahmed Benyahia A, Hajjam A, Talha S, Hajjam M, Andrès E, Hilaire V. E-care: évolution ontologique et amélioration des connaissances pour le suivi des insuffisants cardiaques. Medical Theraphy. 2014;**20**:79-86

[34] Andrès E, Talha S, Hajjam M, Hajjam J, Ervé S, Hajjam A. Experimentation of 2.0 telemedicine in elderly patients with chronic heart failure: A study prospective in 175 patients. European Journal of Internal Medicine. 2018. pii: S0953-6205 (18)30082-7. Doi:10.1016/j. ejim. 2018.02.022. [Epub ahead of print] No abstract available

[35] Mortazavi BJ, Downing NS, Bucholz EM, Dharmarajan K, Manhapra A, Li SX, et al. Analysis of machine learning techniques for heart failure readmissions. Circulation. Cardiovascular Quality and Outcomes. 2016;**9**:629-640

[36] https://www.lesechos.fr/pme-regions/innovateurs/030831110105-plasidia-la-plate-forme-de-telemedecine-personnalisee-pour-les-diabetiques-2128914.php#GfMgmMDeCZSb5mUC.99 [April 2018]

[37] https://www.predimed-technology.fr/ [April 2018]

[38] Charpentier G, Benhamou PY, Dardari D, Clergeot A, Franc S, Schaepelynck-Belicar P, et al. The Diabeo software enabling individualized insulin dose adjustments combined with telemedicine support improves HbA1c in poorly controlled type 1 diabetic patients: A 6-month, randomized, open-label, parallel-group, multicenter trial (tele Diab 1 study). Diabetes Care. 2011;**34**:533-539

Chapter 3

Prevention of Heart Failure

Oleksii Korzh

Additional information is available at the end of the chapter

http://dx.doi.org/10.5772/intechopen.80528

Abstract

Heart failure is a life-threatening disease, and its solution should be seen as a global health priority. Heart failure is indeed a complex disease and has until now been the leading cause of morbidity and mortality in developing and developed countries. Standardized medical therapy was successful in the early stages of heart failure. The advanced stages of heart failure require frequent hospitalization because of the presence of severe heart failure and/or associated comorbid conditions that require the strict implementation of an adequately individualized multidisciplinary approach and quality measures. Even after the development of heart failure, premature deaths can be prevented if they are taught to recognize symptoms and seek immediate medical attention. Public awareness campaigns on these messages have a great potential for improving outcomes for patients with heart failure and, ultimately, for saving lives. It is also quite possible that the prevention of cardiovascular diseases (CVD) in the adult population of the current generation to some extent is only a delay of events or a reduction in mortality from the case, rather than complete prevention. Preventing premature death from cardiovascular disease and years of life adjusted for disability is large but may be due to an increase in the prevalence of cardiovascular disease in the elderly and in very old cases with an epidemic of cardiovascular diseases in the terminal stage, such as chronic heart failure, renal insufficiency, and vascular dementia with all its consequences in terms of greater need for care than for treatment and increased costs of sanitation protection. Continuing research is needed if we want to solve the unmet need for care for patients with heart failure. New methods of treatment are needed for patients with types of heart failure, for which modern treatments ease the symptoms, but do not affect the disease. In the economically developing world, more accessible methods of treatment are desperately needed. International collaborative research on the causes and methods of treating heart failure around the world can benefit tens of millions of people. Compliance with the recommendations of clinical practice is also associated with improved results for patients with heart failure. However, there are significant differences in how closely the doctors follow the recommendations. In order to promote equitable care, improvements should be promoted through the use of indicators and incentives for hospitals that are appropriate to local conditions. To this end, the policy should facilitate the research needed to create an evidence base for performance indicators that reflect improved outcomes for patients.

Keywords: heart failure, prevention, compliance, medical care, lifestyle behaviors

1. Introduction

Cardiovascular disease (CVD) remains the leading cause of death, premature mortality, and disability worldwide. The mortality rate from CVD has been declining since the early 1990s as a result of significant changes in lifestyle and improved health care. This growing prevalence is due to improved survival of people with myocardial infarction and patients with heart failure and a high burden of heart risk factors for people such as hypertension, obesity, diabetes, and smoking. While physical activity and regular exercise are emphasized for the development of general cardiovascular health, modern guidelines for heart failure inadequately emphasized the importance and recommendations for physical activity as a means of preventing a condition [1–3].

Nevertheless, there are certain regions with significantly higher total and mortality from cardiovascular diseases, despite relatively good access to medical care and invasive cardiology procedures. Previous reports conducted among residents of these regions showed adverse lifestyles with a very low prevalence of people who follow current recommendations for the prevention of cardiovascular diseases. This poor adherence to recommended recommendations may be a function of a lack of awareness of the methods of preventing CVD. Several studies have indicated that improving awareness of the risk factors for cardiovascular disease and prevention can be a prerequisite for adopting of a healthy lifestyle [2–5].

To determine the most effective ways to solve the problem of heart failure in different parts of the world, an international approach is needed, as well as the inclusion of necessary measures in everyday practice. Political initiatives at the local, national, and international levels can reduce mortality due to heart failure and improve the quality of life of patients.

2. The global burden of heart failure

In recent years, the survival rates of patients with heart failure have improved in many parts of the world, in parallel with the introduction of modern evidence-based methods and patient management systems. Nevertheless, about 2–17% of those admitted to the hospital with heart failure die in the hospital. Survival rates are better for those who are treated in outpatient clinics, which usually have less pronounced symptoms than those who are treated in the hospital. However, even the newest therapies can only alleviate the symptoms in many patients without slowing the progression of their disease or prolonging life. This is due to the fact that heart failure can arise due to a number of different underlying problems with the structure or function of the heart, some of which are more difficult to treat than others [3, 4].

HF may seriously damage developing countries by creating loss of productivity of cardiac patients. It often severely limits a person's ability to work. Loss of productivity hurts not only

http://dx.doi.org/10.5772/intechopen.80528

the individual but affects the family's income and the country itself by extension. Also, the weakened cardiac patients often need caregivers; consequently, a caregiver often is a family member, and he or she has to stop working in order to nurse a cardiac patient at home. To treat HF and maintain good health in cardiac patients, it is necessary to prescribe several medicines that can be difficult to afford for some people [5–7].

Unfortunately, globalization creates unforeseen problems for most low- and middle-income countries. Adaptation of the western way of life and malnutrition of developed countries are spreading around the world. Limited financial resources and the weak structure of health systems in developing countries pose a barrier to managing the impending global epidemic of chronic diseases. The need to adapt evidence-based treatment plans and model approaches to public health from successful experiences of other countries should become urgent priorities for low- and middle-income countries [8].

Infections remain a common cause of heart failure in many parts of the world and can affect any age. Heart failure is not a disease of the elderly in sub-Saharan Africa, where half of the patients hospitalized with this disease are 55 years or younger. Patients in the Asia-Pacific region are also usually younger than in the western regions. Rheumatic fever due to preventable bacterial infections is an important cause of heart failure in Africa, Asia, Australia, and Latin America. HIV infection is also a major source of cardiovascular disease worldwide. In areas of Latin America where Chagas disease is prevalent, almost half of all cases of heart failure are the direct result of this preventable parasitic infection [9–11].

Heart failure is a widely researched disease because of its burden. There are many studies in which the incidence of heart failure is positively associated with several risk factors. The very first study that addressed the etiology of this disease was a cohort study that followed people for 20 years, a study of the heart of Framingham in the 1970s. According to the Framingham Heart Study, heart failure had several major risk factors. It was found that the highest risk factor for heart failure among the population is hypertension, which accounts for 39% of heart failure in men and 59% in women. The second most significant risk factor was myocardial infarction, which accounts for 34% of heart failure in men and 13% in women. Other important risk factors were diabetes mellitus, left ventricular hypertrophy, and heart valve disease. This was the first scientific evidence of heart failure associated with behavioral factors [12–14].

It has been proven that reducing risk factors will eventually reduce the likelihood of developing heart failure. Most cases of heart failure (90%) are explained by risk factors, such as diabetes, obesity, smoking, blood pressure, and high cholesterol. By reducing BMI, stopping smoking, keeping low cholesterol and blood pressure, and avoiding the other mentioned risk factors, people can potentially be protected from heart failure, cardiovascular diseases, and other chronic diseases. Knowledge of risk factors is very important for the prevention of HF, but they can also be used to combat heart failure and cardiovascular diseases [11, 13–15].

Heart failure significantly affects the quality of life of patients. Fear, anxiety, and depression are common, and work, travel, and everyday social and leisure activities are difficult for people with shortness of breath and extreme fatigue. Emotional, physical, and financial costs are also high for those who care for family members with heart failure. Heart failure leads to a large number of deaths and a widespread disease and requires huge economic and social costs, and the problem worsens. It is time for coordinated awareness programs about heart failure and strategic and policy initiatives to improve patient care.

3. Preventing heart failure in high-risk groups

Prevention of heart failure is of paramount importance. After an establishment the deterioration of a status of the heart can be often treated, but as a rule, it is impossible to cancel. Policymakers should emphasize the need for health professionals in all clinical disciplines to identify patients with diseases that increase the risk of heart failure and prescribe preventive drugs. Ensuring access to preventive drugs should be provided to those who are at greatest risk for developing heart failure, regardless of age, sex, or income. Policymakers should also give priority to the elimination of certain infectious diseases in some parts of the world where they continue to cause heart failure [4, 8, 10].

Risk factors for heart failure vary from lifestyle factors to concomitant diseases, medications, laboratory, and visual characteristics for new biomarkers and genomic markers. The risk of heart failure increases with age, and the male sex is associated with a higher risk. Higher physical activity, increased salt intake, and lower socioeconomic status were associated with increased risk. Hypertension, diabetes, obesity, and coronary disease all increase the risk. More than half of patients hospitalized with heart failure, regardless of the ejection fraction, have coronary artery disease. Hypertension and coronary artery disease are the most common and most powerful risk factors, which bring an increased risk of two to three times. Valvular heart disease increases the risk due to hemodynamic changes.

Obesity, due to a variety of mechanisms, predisposes to heart failure. The excessive use of alcohol increases blood pressure and is a direct myocardial toxin; however, light consumption is moderately associated with risk, especially in men. Smoking contributes to several cardiovascular risk factors associated with heart failure. Dyslipidemia and renal dysfunction predispose to heart failure. Other comorbidities that increase the risk include anemia, sleep breathing disorder, increased heart rate, lung dysfunction, and microalbuminuria. The levels of homocysteine and natriuretic peptide are associated with an increased risk. Serum resistance, lipoproteins associated with phospholipase A2, and myeloperoxidase are also associated with an increased risk [9–12].

Most patients are fragile and elderly with concomitant diseases (e.g., concomitant respiratory diseases and renal dysfunction) that can limit and/or complicate treatment. Although formal classification systems have been developed, the most practical indicator of an increased risk of premature morbidity and mortality or reentering the hospital is the presence of two or more of the following:

- Age ≥ 65 years
- NYHA class III or class IV symptoms
- Charlson Index of Comorbidity Score of 2 or more

http://dx.doi.org/10.5772/intechopen.80528

- Left ventricular ejection fraction (LVEF) ≤ 30%
- Living alone or remote from specialist cardiac services
- Depression
- Language barrier (e.g., non-English speaking)
- Lower socioeconomic status (due to poorer compliance, reduced understanding of reasons for medicines, fewer visits to medical practitioners, high-salt diet in "take-away foods," reduced ability to afford medicines, higher rates of cigarette smoking, etc.)
- Significant renal dysfunction (glomerular filtration rate < 60 mL/min/1.73 m)

Several chemotherapeutic agents, for example, doxorubicin, cyclophosphamide, trastuzumab, and 5-fluorouracil, are associated with heart failure. Inhibitors of cyclooxygenase-2 may increase the risk of myocardial infarction. Thiazolidinediones were associated with edema and heart failure. Several cardiac anatomical and physiological measures are associated with a higher risk, including enlargement of the chamber with an increase in terminal diastolic or terminal systolic dimensions, an increase in left ventricular mass, worsening diastolic filling of the left ventricle, an increase in the left atrium, and asymptomatic systolic dysfunction. There is growing interest in genomic predictors of heart failure.

While patients at high risk benefit greatly from proper and consistent treatment, unfortunately, they often undergo suboptimal management. Their inability to tolerate even minor fluctuations in cardiac and renal function makes them vulnerable to frequent and recurring episodes of acute heart failure.

It is now recognized that up to two-thirds of hospitalizations associated with CHF can be prevented. The following variables are most often associated with poor health outcomes, especially in high-risk patients:

- Inadequate/inappropriate medical or surgical treatment
- Adverse effects of prescribed therapy
- Inadequate knowledge of the underlying illness and prescribed therapy
- Inadequate response to, or recognition of, acute episodes of clinical deterioration
- Nonadherence to prescribed pharmacological treatment
- Lack of motivation/inability to adhere to a non-pharmacological therapy
- Problems with caregivers or extended care facilities
- Inadequate social support

This is especially important for groups at high risk of developing this condition. Many people have diseases that put them at risk of heart failure. Health-care professionals who treat such patients should adopt a broad approach that includes encouraging positive lifestyle changes that reduce the risk of heart failure and prescribe preventive therapy as needed. Medications that control blood pressure, heart rate, and cholesterol levels are effective in preventing heart failure in a large number of people who have conditions such as high blood pressure, coronary heart disease, kidney disease, and diabetes. Pacemakers and the replacement of heart valves can also prevent heart failure in a small number of people who have a particular heart rate or valve disorders. The range of diseases that predispose patients to heart failure is extremely wide. Health-care professionals in all clinical disciplines should receive education to identify patients with diseases that increase the risk of heart failure and prescribe preventive medications. This ensures that as many people as possible get access to therapy [5, 7, 8].

Patients receiving long-term preventive therapy should be evaluated regularly at the expense of health-care providers. In addition, patients with chronic diseases, such as coronary artery disease or Chagas disease, should periodically evaluate and monitor heart changes. Patients with breast cancer are another group that will benefit from such monitoring. Several existing and new methods of treating cancer are toxic to the heart, and it is important for health professionals to be aware of the need to evaluate and manage the risks involved.

Bacterial infections that cause heart disease are largely eliminated in economically developed countries due to the use of antibiotics. In other regions, bacteria and tropical parasites cause a significant proportion of heart failure, many of which can be prevented by appropriate treatment methods. Therefore, the potential benefits of policy initiatives aimed at eliminating infectious diseases extend to preventing heart failure in many parts of the world. In particular, to continue global efforts, it is necessary to eradicate Chagas disease, based on the progress made in Latin America over the past two decades [1, 2].

Preventive treatment could be started earlier, identifying people with early signs of abnormal cardiac muscle remodeling. Unfortunately, large-scale screening programs, such as those that allowed earlier treatment of bowel cancer, cervical cancer, and breast cancer, are unfortunately not possible, because there is no simple diagnostic test for heart failure. Early changes in the structure or function of the heart can be detected using medical imaging technology; however, it is inadvisable to perform these complex procedures in a large number of people with diseases that lead to heart failure and, of course, not for the general population. In the future, extended genetic tests and statistical modeling of risk groups that take into account the myriad potential causes of heart failure may be available, and this can allow individuals to be identified for in-depth screening.

Targeting preventive drugs to people with the highest risk of heart failure can increase profitability, allowing more people to take advantage. Further research in these areas continues and should continue to be supported by public and private funds. In addition, information programs should be directed at everyone who has medical conditions that predispose to heart failure. They should include education about the symptoms of heart failure and the benefits of positive lifestyle changes. The same messages are important for public information programs [3–6].

Preventing heart failure in the elderly is becoming a more urgent health priority, as the age of the population. Heart failure is the most common cause of hospitalization in people older than 65 years in economically developed regions. Elderly patients hospitalized with heart failure mostly are women. Although a number of studies of patients with heart failure have shown that survival rates are better in women than in men, recent studies have shown that long-term prospects for women are not as good as previously thought. Therefore, initiatives aimed at improving the prevention of heart failure should include strategies to reach older people, especially older women [14–16].

In economically developed countries, heart failure is more common and most likely the cause of death in people with low socioeconomic status than the rest of the population. This is still the case after adjusting for age differences, the use of drugs, and the proportion of people with other cardiac diseases. The view was expressed that the role of housing can be played by housing stability, social support, substance abuse, language skills, and distance to the hospital.

Several studies have reported a reduction in the risk of heart failure with a healthy lifestyle. It has been shown that healthy weight, avoidance of smoking, exercise, and healthy eating reduce the risk factors for heart failure, including ischemic disease, diabetes, and hypertension. Recently, researchers in the health research of doctors reported that habits of a healthy lifestyle, that is, normal body weight, rather than smoking, regular exercise, moderate alcohol consumption, consumption of breakfast cereals, and consumption of fruits and vegetables, were associated with a lower risk of heart disease with the most high risk of 21.3% in men who do not observe any of these habits and the lowest risk of 10.1% in men who adhere to 4 or more of them.

4. Healthy lifestyle, behavior, and socioeconomic issues

Although many heart failure risk factors have been described, determining their role in predicting a future event is still difficult. Despite a strong etiological relationship to the disease, the risk factor may be limited in its prognostic role. Although individual risk factors for heart failure, such as hypertension, are well described, how do we clearly identify individual risk in patients with different combinations of risk factors? For coronary events, schemes for predicting multiple risks have been developed, for example, the Framingham risk score. However, heart failure syndrome is a spectrum from ischemic to nonischemic etiology and from normal to depressed ejection fraction. Older patients may develop heart failure due to age-related cardiovascular changes in the absence of traditional risk factors. Thus, high-risk subjects cannot be detected using coronary risk regimes [15].

Several unique problems make the assessment of the risk of heart failure difficult. First, heart failure is a clinical diagnosis, and this leads to a variety of opinions and diagnostic uncertainties in a number of cases. The most common clinical criteria used to diagnose heart failure are the Framingham criteria, which require at least two basic or one basic and two lower criteria. The main criteria include paroxysmal nocturnal dyspnea, a dilated vein in the throat, rales, radiographic cardiomegaly, acute pulmonary edema, gallop S3, increased venous pressure > 16 cm H_2O, circulation time ≥ 25 seconds, hepatojugular reflux or pulmonary edema, or visceral cluster or cardiomegaly at the autopsy. Minor criteria included bilateral ankle edema, night cough, shortness of breath with normal tension, hepatomegaly, pleural effusion, a decrease in vital capacity by one-third of the maximum, and heart rate ≥ 120 beats per minute. Researchers from the cardiovascular study have developed alternative criteria that included the use of drugs and imaging techniques. When both sets of criteria were compared, only half of the patients were considered to have heart failure by both criteria, while the other half were labeled either one or the other, but not both. A similar discrepancy was shown between diagnoses of administrative categories compared to a detailed overview of the diagram [2, 13–16].

Social changes can affect the CVD epidemic in different ways. It may be influenced by globalization, migration, socioeconomic changes, and unemployment. Over the years, differences in the incidence of CVD among countries, regions, and areas have increased; these inequalities can be explained by the components of human behavior, such as diet, exercise, smoking, and work-related functions, as well as overcrowding, unemployment, and other deprivation indicators. The expected life expectancy is constantly increasing with income.

5. Smoking of tobacco

Smoking is a strong predictor of heart failure in men and women; 45% and 88% have an increased risk. The harmful effect of tobacco, apparently, does not depend on the form of use. An increased risk of cardiovascular disease is reported when tobacco is used by non-smokers. There is no "safe" level of smoking; a single cigarette can strengthen the left ventricle, and only one to four cigarettes a day double the risk of myocardial infarction. Mechanisms leading to heart failure in smokers include (i) indirect effects, that is, causing or exacerbating associated diseases associated with heart failure, and (ii) direct exposure to the myocardium.

Tobacco smoking remains one of the most important preventable causes of premature mortality, and quitting is the most cost-effective strategy for the prevention of cardiovascular disease. Improvements have been made with regard to tobacco smoking, in some countries more than in others, with large differences in accordance with the socioeconomic class. Governmental constraints and rules were successful; high taxes on tobacco products are the most effective policy measure to reduce smoking among young people. However, this needs to be complemented by continuing campaigns in the field of health education, especially those targeting young people and other subgroups of society. There must be restrictions on advertising, promotion, and sponsorship by the industry [12, 16].

All smokers should be advised to quit. Patients should be referred to formal programs to discontinue therapy, and pharmacological therapy should be offered to increase success. Current recommended strategies include the following: (a) Medicines. Several drugs are available for tobacco dependence. Seven first-line drugs significantly increase long-term rates of abstinence from smoking, including bupropion SR, nicotinic gum or inhaler or cake or nasal spray, or patch and varenicline. (b) Counseling and psychosocial support. Individual, group, and telephone practical consultations and social support are effective, and their effectiveness increases with the intensity of treatment. (c) Combination. However, the combination of counseling and medication is more effective than one, so clinicians should encourage all people who attempt to stop using both counseling and medication.

http://dx.doi.org/10.5772/intechopen.80528

Smokers who want to quit smoking should get professional help if needed. Short interventions with recommendations for cessation of smoking, together with pharmacological support and follow-up visits, are effective and safe, but not enough, even for smokers with established ischemic heart disease. If the smoker is ready to stop, a termination plan should be prepared, including the release date, information for friends and families asking for support, and removing all tobacco and smoking-related items from the immediate environment and, finally, ideally within a month and every month after that for 4 months. On a subsequent visit, a person should be congratulated if he/she has stopped smoking. In case of relapse, a more intensive approach should be considered, for example, referral of a specialist or center for cessation of smoking. Avoidance of secondhand smoke is another important recommendation for CVD prevention.

If the recommendations, stimulation, and motivation are likely to be insufficient, drug therapy should be considered at an early stage, including nicotine replacement therapy (NRT), bupropion, or varenicline. Pharmacotherapy for smoking cessation can double or triple throw rates, and a combination of pharmacotherapy and counseling improves throw rates.

The success of cessation of smoking with varenicline is higher than with bupropion; varenicline doubles the chances of stopping smoking compared to placebo. Varenicline reduces cravings for cigarettes and withdrawal symptoms; it should be run 1 to 2 weeks before the release date. Hypersensitivity is the only contraindication. Nausea is the most common side effect, especially at the beginning of therapy and if taken with food. In some cases, a dose titration may be required.

Electronic cigarettes, or e-cigarettes, can deliver high concentrations of nicotine as a vapor and have been recommended as a measure to help stop smoking conventional cigarettes. The results of studies of the cardiovascular effect of electronic cigarettes are inconsistent, but in some cases, an increased risk is documented.

6. Dietary habits

As for the dietary habits of the population, the changes occurred in different areas. For example, consumption of salt and saturated fats has been reduced in most societies. The food industry has reduced the presence of trans-fatty acids in different foods. This was promoted by regulatory initiatives in some communities. Nevertheless, the potential for preventing cardiovascular disease through dietary adaptations is still poorly implemented. Compliance with a balanced diet is usually limited. Control of high blood pressure, dyslipidemia, and dysglycemia can be significantly improved due to lifestyle changes. Achieving better adherence to dietary recommendations requires an understanding of the determinants of poor compliance. At the population level, structural measures, such as product information and user-friendly food labeling, can improve health-friendly options. Energy-intensive products with nutrient deficiencies are usually highly available and inexpensive; marketing of such products may be limited and taxed.

In the diet "Dietary Approaches to Stopping Hypertension" (DASH), people are encouraged to consume more (i) fruits and vegetables; (ii) grains and cereals; (iii) lean meat, fish, and poultry; (iv) low-fat or low-fat dairy products; and (v) nuts, seeds, and pulses and reduce consumption of red meat, fat, and sugar while maintaining low-sodium intake. Initially it was elevated for hypertension; however, recent data confirm a reduction in the risk of heart failure with an observed decrease of 37% in women who adhere to the DASH diet. The DASH diet can help prevent heart failure by lowering blood pressure and coronary heart disease. Daily consumption of whole grain breakfast cereals was associated with a 30% reduction in heart failure, egg consumption more than twice a day was associated with an increase of 64%, fish consumption was associated with a 20–31% lower heart failure rate depending on consumption, and consumption of 100 mmol or more of sodium was associated with a 26% rate; only the consumption of nuts was not associated with heart failure. Whole grains can protect against the risk of heart failure as a result of exposure to weight, hypertension, myocardial infarction, and diabetes mellitus.

Fish consumption has a beneficial effect on the risk of heart failure with about 20% less risk associated with consumption one to two times a week and about 30% less risk when consumed ≥3 times a week, compared with consumption less than one time per week/month. The estimated consumption of marine n-3 fatty acids was associated with a 37% reduction in the risk of heart failure in the highest quintile of consumption compared to the lowest. Short-term tests of fish oil supplementation of 3–5 g per day can reduce the risk, while dietary doses of about 0.5 g per day can lead to more modest effects, which over time can reduce the risk of heart failure. It has been reported that the consumption of fried fish or baked fish is inversely related to systolic blood pressure, C-reactive protein level, and carotid intimal medial thickness, while consumption of fried fish is positively associated with them, indicating that the type of preparation can influence the effects.

At the clinical level, general practitioners have the opportunity to provide advice on a diet for treating risk factors for coronary diseases. However, obstacles related to time constraints, knowledge, and perceived effectiveness were reported. The degree to which doctors are familiar with a healthy dietary pattern (i.e., DASH, the Mediterranean diet) and with the translation of this information into practical recommendations may be limited. A multidisciplinary approach, including dieticians and nutritionists, can help but needs to improve coverage of reimbursement.

At the individual level, new strategies can help improve patient self-control and lead to a sustained behavior change. Many applications and devices are available that provide data that can be useful for lifestyle changes and patient self-care.

7. Physical activity

Physical inactivity is an important risk factor for cardiovascular disease, including heart failure. Regular physical activity has important and broad benefits, such as reducing the risk of cardiovascular disease, hypertension, and diabetes. Physical activity is a key to good health and an important component of weight loss and weight maintenance, improving the profile of lipoproteins and reducing the risk of hypertension, diabetes, and coronary artery disease. These favorable effects on the profile of cardiovascular risks, in turn, reduce the likelihood of heart failure [14–16].

http://dx.doi.org/10.5772/intechopen.80528

Promotion of physical exercises is a crucial and central issue in all strategies for the prevention of cardiovascular diseases. At the individual level, physical activity should be recommended at different times; he must become part of ordinary life from childhood. Children and adolescents should be encouraged to spend from 30 to 45 minutes of exercise at school or in their free time every day. This should be maintained as long as possible, through adolescence to adulthood.

Physical activity can also reduce left ventricular hypertrophy and improve endothelial function. Chronic physical activity reduces the production of cytokines by fat tissue, skeletal muscles, and endothelial and blood mononuclear cells and regulates antioxidant enzymes. These modifying effects on risk factors for heart failure or the intermediate pathways leading to heart failure can reduce heart failure. Integration of physical activity into everyday life of the population proved to be a difficult task.

Healthy adults in all age groups are encouraged to choose pleasant physical exercises that fit into everyday life on most days of the week. It is recommended to perform at least 150 minutes per week of moderate aerobic physical activity (30 minutes for 5 days a week) or 75 minutes per week of intense aerobic physical activity (15 minutes for 5 days a week) or a combination thereof. At the individual level, the purpose of the exercise should be more personalized. Therefore, a brief history of the individual's physical level is needed (how many minutes per day is spent on average with activity at moderate or strong intensity).

Currently, the recommendations of the American College of Sports Medicine and the American Heart Association for regular physical activity in healthy adults 18–65 years include the following: (a) Aerobic activity. Aerobic physical activity with moderate intensity for at least 30 minutes for 5 days a week or intense aerobic activity for a minimum of 20 minutes for 3 days a week. (b) Strengthening of muscles. It is recommended that 8–10 exercises are performed for 2 or several days without Monday to a week using the main muscle groups. To maximize the development of strength, you should use resistance (weight), which allows you to perform 8–12 repetitions of each exercise, which leads to strong-willed fatigue. (c) Dose of activity. Activity of intensive intensity can have a greater benefit than physical activity of medium intensity.

Walks have been reported as useful for primary prevention; this should be done by individuals who do not adhere to current recommendations.

Based on this and taking into account the individual choice, it is possible to give advice on the most appropriate activities, on how to move forward, about what goals should be set to achieve and maintain health benefits from active lifestyles. It is necessary to identify barriers to achieving a more active lifestyle, perceived by the individual, and to explore ways of overcoming them. For people at work, it is recommended to recommend an active trip, as well as active breaks from long periods of sitting. In people who are not able to perform a minimum, or in inactive subjects who are just beginning to engage in any activity, even the lowest recommended level should be recommended. It should be emphasized that any increase in activity will be associated with a beneficial health impact, even before the learning effect becomes apparent, and that it is normal for gradual work for any given purpose.

7.1. Overweight and obesity

There are several plausible mechanisms for the association of obesity and an increased risk of heart failure. Indirect but well-known and documented mechanism is the effect of obesity in heart failure with the help of other risk factors. The increase in BMI is a risk factor for the development of hypertension, diabetes mellitus, and dyslipidemia, all of which increase the risk of myocardial infarction, which is an important precursor of heart failure. In addition, hypertension and diabetes mellitus independently increase the risk of HF occurrence. It has also been shown that increased BMI is associated with altered left ventricular remodeling, possibly due to increased hemodynamic loading, neurohormonal activation, and increased oxidative stress. Studies have shown that obesity can have a direct effect on the myocardium, demonstrating a loss of cardiac function through cardiac steatosis and lipoapoptosis.

The body mass index is associated with heart failure in a positive and linear way in both sexes. Although the body mass index in the obesity area ($\geq$30 kg/m^2) is clearly associated with an increased risk of heart failure, there are disputes regarding the body mass index in the overweight range (25–29.9 kg/m^2). However, recent data confirm that overweight is also associated with heart failure. Abdominal obesity may be a stronger predictor of heart failure than complete obesity, even in the absence of coronary heart disease. Several mechanisms have been proposed that increase the body mass index, the risk of heart failure, including (a) changes in the cardiac load, (b) changes in cardiac structure and function, (c) activation of neurohumoral and inflammatory pathways, (d) promotion of atherogenic conditions, (e) a predisposition to breathing with sleep disorders, and (f) a chronic kidney disease.

Although elevated BMI is well known as a risk factor for heart failure, this study showed that an elevated BMI is not a risk factor for increasing mortality but rather is associated with a trend toward improved survival. This counterintuitive epidemiological link between survival outcomes and traditional risk factors is called reverse epidemiology or "paradoxical obesity," and it is now well documented in numerous studies and in the literature on heart failure.

The exact mechanisms underlying the paradox of obesity have not been clearly defined. There are several theories. A common explanation for the increase in survival in obese patients with heart failure is that additional fatty tissue provides greater reserves against catabolic changes associated with the disease process that can lead to cardiac cachexia. Cardiac cachexia is a syndrome that includes progressive weight loss and changes in the body composition, which carries a destructive prognosis for heart failure, as well as in other painful conditions.

The basic approach to risk reduction for obese patients should include weight control and physical activity, as well as control of related risk factors such as hypertension, diabetes, sleep disorders, and metabolic syndrome components. Changes in the myocardium with nonsurgical or surgical weight loss are possible, and a slight weight loss is effective; weight loss of 10% reduces systolic dysfunction, and a weight loss of 8–10 kg leads to a significant decrease in the size of the left ventricle and the mass index and improves diastolic function. Significant weight loss reduces the thickness and volume of the wall of the left ventricle, filling pressure, improves diastolic parameters, and improves systolic function of the left ventricle. The role of metabolic and neurohumoral modification may take precedence over hemodynamic effects, since left ventricular mass or functional improvement occurs independently of load changes.

http://dx.doi.org/10.5772/intechopen.80528

7.2. Alcohol consumption

Although epidemiological data constantly demonstrate the harmful effects on health associated with alcohol use, current literature cites some evidence of reducing the risk of heart failure with mild and moderate alcohol consumption. However, in order to fully understand the relationship between mild to moderate alcohol consumption and heart failure, several gaps need to be filled, especially the role of alcohol samples, beverage types, and genetic variations affecting alcohol metabolism and the effect of light on moderate drinking in predicting mortality and concomitant morbidity among people with heart failure. In the absence of large randomized studies of moderate alcohol consumption and heart failure, residual mixing or immeasurable confusion cannot be ruled out as possible explanations of the observed relationships. Thus, for patients who do not consume alcohol, it would be premature to recommend mild to moderate alcohol consumption as a means to reduce the risk of HF, given the possible risk of abuse and the resulting consequences.

Excessive consumption of alcohol is associated with alcoholic cardiomyopathy. Interestingly, other data are consistent with the possible benefits of moderate alcohol consumption for the risk of heart failure. In addition, it was reported that mild to moderate alcohol consumption is associated with a 40–50% lower risk of heart failure than with a previous myocardial infarction, whereas in the same study, the risk of heart failure without previous myocardial infarction among people who use heavy drinks was 1.7 times higher than that of abstained. Similar results were presented in the study of the health of doctors. The favorable effects of alcohol on the risk of developing hypertension, myocardial infarction, and diabetes mellitus have also been reported, while alcohol increases the level of high-density lipoprotein cholesterol, increases insulin sensitivity, reduces the level of inflammatory markers and clotting factors in plasma, and increases the level of adiponectin.

8. Management of cardiovascular risk factors

All current guidelines on the prevention of CVD in clinical practice recommend the assessment of total CVD risk because atherosclerotic CVD is usually the product of a number of risk factors. Prevention of CVD in a given person should be adapted to his or her total CVD risk: the higher the risk, the more intensive the action should be. The stratification of the community into different levels of total CVD risk was given in recent guidelines.

8.1. Dyslipidemias

The treatment goals for LDL-C depend on the total CVD risk of the patient and of the baseline LDL-C level. In patients at very high CVD risk, an LDL-C goal of <1.8 mmol/L (70 mg/dL), or a reduction of at least 50% if the baseline LDL-C level is between 1.8 and 3.5 mmol/L (70 and 135 mg/dL), is recommended.

In patients at high CVD risk, an LDL-C goal of <2.6 mmol/L (100 mg/dL), or a reduction of at least 50% if the baseline LDL-C level is between 2.6 and 5.2 mmol/L (100 and 200 mg/dL), is recommended. In subjects at moderate risk, an LDL-C goal of <3.0 mmol/L (115 mg/dL) should be considered.

Statins have proven effective in patients with coronary heart disease; however, their usefulness in staging left ventricular dysfunction remains under investigation. The role of statins in the prevention of heart failure is shown.

Based on the results of the IMPROVE-IT study, further reduction in LDL-C by the addition of ezetimibe should be considered in patients with cardiovascular diseases with LDL-C ≥ 70 mg/dl (≥1.8 mmol/L), despite the maximum allowable dose of statin. Now a new family of drugs that lower lipid levels is available. These inhibitors of subtilisin/kexin type 9 retardate convertase (PCSK9) further reduce LDL-C in addition to what can be achieved with statins. In a FOURIER study, inhibition of PCSK9 with evolocumab against statins lowered LDL-C to a median of 30 mg/dL (0.78 mmol/L) and reduced cardiovascular events. The use of this drug should be considered in patients with a very high risk of cardiovascular disease, in which LDL-C remains elevated, despite the fact that it is treated with a maximum dose of statins in combination with ezetimibe or in patients with statin intolerance.

8.2. Arterial hypertension

Elevated blood pressure (BP) is one of the most powerful modifiable risk factors for cardiovascular disease. The beneficial effects of lowering blood pressure on the reduction of stroke, myocardial infarction, heart failure, and death have been shown in numerous RCTs and in various meta-analyses. BP reduction can be achieved through lifestyle changes and drug therapy [17–19].

Progression progresses from hypertension to structural changes in the ventricles and systolic and diastolic ventricular dysfunction. The increase in chronic load, left ventricular mass, and stress, accompanied by a deterioration in the properties of diastolic filling, occurs in a chronic environment. Disproportionately increased left ventricular mass leads to inadequate microcirculation for perfusion of the hypertrophied myocardium, which leads to subendocardial hypoperfusion, ischemia. These changes increase the risk of developing coronary thrombosis and a heart attack characterized by loss of contractile function, neurohormonal activation, and ventricular remodeling, which leads to the development of systolic dysfunction. Anomalies in neurohormonal activation and the balance of water and electrolyte also play a role in the cascade, which leads to hypertension to heart failure [20–22].

8.3. Dysglycemia and diabetes mellitus

In people with impaired glucose tolerance, the development of type 2 diabetes mellitus (DM) can be delayed or prevented. In patients with type 2 diabetes, cardiovascular disease can be prevented by good control of risk factors for cardiovascular disease. Intensive management of hyperglycemia also reduces the risk of microvascular complications.

Diabetes mellitus is an independent risk factor for heart failure in all age groups. The relative risk of heart failure in patients with diabetes varies from 1.3 to 2.7, increasing to 4 in patients under the age of 65 and 11 in individuals younger than 45 years. Several mechanisms have been proposed to explain the increased risk. Combinations associated with heart failure, including obesity, hypertension, and coronary artery disease, are common among people

http://dx.doi.org/10.5772/intechopen.80528

with diabetes. Insulin resistance itself can cause disturbances in the cardiac structure and function [23–25].

Unfortunately, the prevalence of type 2 DM increases in most parts of the world, mainly because of unbalanced diets and lack of physical activity. The diagnosis of DM is also problematic in a large number of people and even in patients with established CVD. Screening should be considered by evaluating HbA1c or fasting blood glucose levels. When there is any doubt, you should offer a test for glucose tolerance orally.

For most nonpregnant adults with type 1 or type 2 DM, it is recommended to reduce HbA1c < 7.0% (<53 mmol / mol) to reduce the risk of cardiovascular disease and the risk of microvascular complications. When diagnosed or at the beginning of a DM, the target HbA1c ≤ 6.5% (≤48 mmol/mol) should be considered in patients who are not brittle and do not have CVD.

Metformin is recommended as first-line therapy if it is tolerated and not contraindicated after assessing kidney function. In patients with diabetes and cardiovascular disease, the use of sodium glucose-based cotransporter-2 (SGCT2) inhibitors reduced cardiovascular and total mortality without significant adverse effects. These drugs should be considered at an early stage of treatment of DM in these patients. Optimal management of LDL-C and BP levels is of great importance for all patients with DM [3, 24, 25].

8.4. Public awareness of heart failure and compliance

Appropriate care for heart failure and adequate provision of care and research require recognition of its clinical, social, and economic importance not only by health authorities and providers of health services but also by the general public. Without recognition of the symptoms and their severity, people with heart failure will not seek immediate treatment—patients often present with a long history of dyspnea. Awareness of the causes of HF can help to make appropriate lifestyle changes to reduce the risk. In addition, awareness of the benefits of treatment can help compliance and encourage patients to seek appropriate care. However, there is a lack of information about public awareness of HF. Studies have shown a relatively low understanding and treatment of heart failure by general practitioners. If doctors are not aware of the importance of HF, it is unlikely that the general public will have a good understanding [26–28].

A large number of premature deaths are due to ignorance of the causes and symptoms of heart failure. There is an urgent need for public information programs that determine heart failure in a simple and accessible language, explain how to recognize symptoms, and stress the need for emergency medical care. Other important messages are that most types of heart failure can be prevented and a healthy lifestyle can reduce the risk. Policymakers should support the development and implementation of public awareness programs targeted at these messages. The public understanding of the symptoms of heart failure is dangerously low.

Cost-effective information, education, and support programs to reduce the risk of heart failure should be at the forefront of public health guidelines. Lifestyle events can have a significant impact on the health of the world, because obesity, diabetes, cigarette smoking, and high blood pressure significantly increase the likelihood of heart failure. Renewing commitment to public education, the importance of healthy nutrition and weight, regular exercise, and prevention of smoking should be a priority for policymakers [29, 30].

In low- and middle-income countries, lifestyle-based measures to prevent heart failure were calculated as more cost-effective than pharmaceutical interventions. The acute need to take risks into life throughout the world is recognized by the United Nations, including in regions such as sub-Saharan Africa, where noncommunicable diseases associated with western lifestyles are not yet the leading causes of death or disease. Given the increasing number of patients with heart failure in economically developing regions, governments should be encouraged to combine lifestyle-based preventive measures with their programs to combat hunger and the epidemic. One could consider the issue of regulating aggressive marketing of high-calorie foods by large global corporate enterprises, especially schoolchildren and adolescents [31–33].

Compliance with the recommendations of clinical practice is often associated with improved outcomes for patients with heart failure. However, in many countries there are significant differences in how closely hospitals follow the recommendations of national recommendations for heart failure. In response, policymakers must protect the fairness of care for all patients. First, it is important to promote heart failure training programs that raise awareness of the guidelines among all relevant health professionals. Secondly, better care should be encouraged, using performance indicators and incentives appropriate to local conditions. Funding is needed to research evidence-based health-care performance indicators that reflect improvements in clinical outcomes for patients with heart failure. By improving health care, policymakers can provide a health system that provides timely access to the diagnosis and treatment of heart failure and then a consistent transition to long-term management.

Diagnosis of heart failure can be difficult, even for skilled professionals. Not all patients with heart failure have typical symptoms, and the same symptoms can be experienced by patients who do not have heart failure. For an accurate diagnosis, a number of diagnostic tools and information are required in combination with clinical judgment and expert knowledge.

Many patients initially do not see an expert in heart failure due to the fact that they are part of the health-care system. Those with severe symptoms, such as dyspnea at rest, are most often evaluated by paramedics or emergency doctors in the hospital, whereas those with less obvious life-threatening symptoms are more likely to go to their family doctor or outpatient clinic. Educational programs are needed to raise awareness about clinical practice recommendations among health professionals from a wide range of specialties that may be the first to encounter patients with undiagnosed heart failure.

Recommendations for the use of drugs for the treatment of heart failure are based on clinical trials conducted mainly in Europe and the United States. In other parts of the world, the underlying causes of heart failure are different, and it is not safe to assume that drugs will be equally effective in all patient groups. A further clinical study to investigate the efficacy of treating heart failure in different patient groups around the world should be maintained [32–34].

The world survey showed the need to improve patients' self-care. Most patients reported taking medication as prescribed, but few reported having control of their weight or regular training. Educational programs are a priority, but they need to be developed carefully, because it is reported that patients with a deeper knowledge of heart failure are more likely to delay treatment. This may reflect false optimism and a lack of understanding that controlling the symptoms of heart failure does not slow the progression of the disease. The learning environment should also be carefully considered. Short video clips, text messages, and social networks can be used to deliver simple but accurate messages. Currently, according to estimates, 6 billion people own a mobile phone; technology can be an important way to reach remote and socially economically disadvantaged [27–31].

Teaching people how to support a partner, family member, or friend with heart failure is also an important part of encouraging self-help. Patients are more likely to engage in useful self-help if they have someone who will help them than if they were socially isolated. This emphasizes the need to improve support for communities of socioeconomically disadvantaged patients and those who live alone. Policymakers should provide resources to educate and support people with heart failure and their caregivers, allowing them to actively engage in long-term care.

9. Conclusion

Prevention of disease and death due to heart failure should be a priority in the field of health. Despite the increasing number of people living and dying of heart failure, awareness of this disease is low among the public, politicians, and even some health professionals. Despite the lack of treatment for heart failure, many cases can be prevented, and most patients can effectively be treated to improve quality of life and survival. Policymakers are responsible for ensuring that as many people as possible can take advantage of affordable prevention, diagnosis, treatment, and long-term treatment of heart failure. At the same time, research should be supported in areas where immediate unmet needs exist.

All current recommendations for the prevention of cardiovascular disease in clinical practice recommend an estimate of the overall risk of cardiovascular disease, since atherosclerotic cardiovascular risk is usually the result of a number of risk factors. Prevention of cardiovascular disease in this person should be adapted to his or her overall risk of cardiovascular disease: the higher the risk, the more intense the action should be.

The positive impact of specialized management programs on survival suggests that these factors also lead to a significant number of preventable deaths. Many of the factors listed above are often considered in "normal conditions" of clinical trials with increased monitoring and individualized observation. It is therefore not surprising that patients in clinical trials usually have lower than expected morbidity and mortality rates.

Any program aimed at improving long-term management must recognize that patients with heart failure play a key role in their own care. Self-service includes maintenance, monitoring, and management. Maintenance involves taking medication as prescribed, regular meals, and a healthy diet. Monitoring involves monitoring of symptoms and weight (which can serve as a warning sign of increasing fluid accumulation). Management involves responding to changes in symptoms by adjusting the doses of certain drugs if they are prescribed for "use as needed" (e.g., drugs that increase urine production to reduce fluid accumulation) or by seeking medical help if symptoms worsen.

Author details

Oleksii Korzh

Address all correspondence to: okorzh2007@gmail.com

Department of General Practice-Family Medicine, Kharkiv Medical Academy of Postgraduate Education, Kharkiv, Ukraine

References

[1] Robertson J, McElduff P, Pearson SA, et al. The health services burden of heart failure: An analysis using linked population health data-sets. BMC Health Services Research. 2012;**12**:103. DOI: 10.1186/1472-6963-12-103

[2] Sato N, Kajimoto K, Keida T, et al. Clinical features and outcome in hospitalized heart failure in Japan (from the ATTEND registry). Circulation Journal. 2013;**77**:944-951

[3] Cleland JG, Swedberg K, Follath F, et al. The EuroHeart failure survey programme—A survey on the quality of care among patients with heart failure in Europe. Part 1: Patient characteristics and diagnosis. European Heart Journal. 2003;**24**:442-463

[4] AlHabib KF, Elasfar AA, Alfaleh H et al. Clinical features, management, and short- and long-term outcomes of patients with acute decompensated heart failure: Phase I results of the HEARTS database. European Journal of Heart Failure. 2014: DOI: 10.1002/ejhf.57

[5] Roger VL, Weston SA, Redfield MM, et al. Trends in heart failure incidence and survival in a community-based population. Journal of the American Medical Association. 2004;**292**:344-350

[6] Huelsmann M, Neuhold S, Resl M, et al. PONTIAC (NT-proBNP selected prevention of cardiac events in a population of diabetic patients without a history of cardiac disease): A prospective randomized controlled trial. Journal of the American College of Cardiology. 2013;**62**:1365-1372

[7] Ledwidge M, Gallagher J, Conlon C, et al. Natriuretic peptide-based screening and collaborative care for heart failure: The STOP-HF randomized trial. Journal of the American Medical Association. 2013;**310**:66-74

[8] Felker GM, Hasselblad V, Hernandez AF, et al. Biomarker-guided therapy in chronic heart failure: A meta-analysis of randomized controlled trials. American Heart Journal. 2009;**158**:422-430

[9] Persson H, Erntell H, Eriksson B, et al. Improved pharmacological therapy of chronic heart failure in primary care: A randomized study of NT-proBNP guided management of heart failure—SIGNAL-HF (Swedish Intervention study—Guidelines and NT-proBNP AnaLysis in Heart Failure). European Journal of Heart Failure. 2010;**12**:1300-1308

[10] Shah MR, Califf RM, Nohria A, et al. The STARBRITE trial: A randomized, pilot study of B-type natriuretic peptide-guided therapy in patients with advanced heart failure. Journal of Cardiac Failure. 2011;**17**:613-621

[11] Gaggin HK, Mohammed AA, Bhardwaj A, et al. Heart failure outcomes and benefits of NT-proBNP-guided management in the elderly: Results from the prospective, randomized ProBNP outpatient tailored chronic heart failure therapy (PROTECT) study. Journal of Cardiac Failure. 2012;**18**:626-634

[12] O'Connor CM, Hasselblad V, Mehta RH, et al. Triage after hospitalization with advanced heart failure: The ESCAPE (Evaluation Study of Congestive Heart Failure and Pulmonary Artery Catheterization Effectiveness) risk model and discharge score. Journal of the American College of Cardiology. 2010;**55**:872-878

[13] Kociol RD, McNulty SE, Hernandez AF, et al. Markers of decongestion, dyspnea relief, and clinical outcomes among patients hospitalized with acute heart failure. Circulation: Heart Failure. 2013;**6**:240-245

[14] Son CS, Kim YN, Kim HS, et al. Decision-making model for early diagnosis of congestive heart failure using rough set and decision tree approaches. Journal of Biomedical Informatics. 2012;**45**:999-1008

[15] Kelder JC, Cramer MJ, Van WJ, et al. The diagnostic value of physical examination and additional testing in primary care patients with suspected heart failure. Circulation. 2011;**124**:2865-2873

[16] Zairis MN, Tsiaousis GZ, Georgilas AT, et al. Multimarker strategy for the prediction of 31 days cardiac death in patients with acutely decompensated chronic heart failure. International Journal of Cardiology. 2010;**141**:284-290

[17] McMurray JJV, Packer M, Desai AS, et al. Angiotensin-neprilysin inhibition versus enalapril in heart failure. The New England Journal of Medicine. 2014;**371**:993-1004

[18] Yusuf S, Teo KK, Pogue J, et al. Telmisartan, ramipril, or both in patients at high risk for vascular events. The New England Journal of Medicine. 2008;**358**:1547-1559

[19] Yusuf S, Teo K, Anderson C, et al. Effects of the angiotensin-receptor blocker telmisartan on cardiovascular events in high-risk patients intolerant to angiotensin-converting enzyme inhibitors: A randomised controlled trial. Lancet. 2008;**372**:1174-1183

[20] Sakata Y, Shiba N, Takahashi J, et al. Clinical impacts of additive use of olmesartan in hypertensive patients with chronic heart failure: The supplemental benefit of an angiotensin receptor blocker in hypertensive patients with stable heart failure using olmesartan (SUPPORT) trial. European Heart Journal. 2015;**36**:915-923

[21] Eschalier R, McMurray JJV, Swedberg K, et al. Safety and efficacy of eplerenone in patients at high risk for hyperkalemia and/or worsening renal function: Analyses of the EMPHASIS-HF study subgroups (Eplerenone in Mild Patients Hospitalization and SurvIval Study in Heart Failure). Journal of the American College of Cardiology. 2013;**62**:1585-1593

[22] Rouleau JL, Pfeffer MA, Stewart DJ, et al. Comparison of vasopeptidase inhibitor, omapatrilat, and lisinopril on exercise tolerance and morbidity in patients with heart failure: IMPRESS randomised trial. Lancet. 2000;**356**:615-620

[23] Bohm M, Robertson M, Ford I, et al. Influence of cardiovascular and noncardiovascular co-morbidities on outcomes and treatment effect of heart rate reduction with ivabradine in stable heart failure (from the SHIFT Trial). American Journal of Cardiology. 2015;**116**: 1890-1897

[24] Piller LB, Baraniuk S, Simpson LM, et al. Long-term follow-up of participants with heart failure in the antihypertensive and lipid-lowering treatment to prevent heart attack trial (ALLHAT). Circulation. 2011;**124**:1811-1818

[25] Kostis JB, Davis BR, Cutler J, et al. Prevention of heart failure by antihypertensive drug treatment in older persons with isolated systolic hypertension. SHEP Cooperative Research Group. Journal of the American Medical Association. 1997;**278**:212-216

[26] Xie X, Atkins E, Lv J, et al. Effects of intensive blood pressure lowering on cardiovascular and renal outcomes: Updated systematic review and meta-analysis. Lancet. 2016;**387**:435-443

[27] Heidenreich PA, Hernandez AF, Yancy CW, et al. Get with the guidelines program participation, process of care, and outcome for medicare patients hospitalized with heart failure. Circulation. Cardiovascular Quality and Outcomes. 2012;**5**:37-43

[28] Butler J, Fonarow GC, Gheorghiade M. Need for increased awareness and evidence-based therapies for patients hospitalized for heart failure. Journal of the American Medical Association. 2013;**310**:2035-2036

[29] Palaniswamy C, Mishkin A, Aronow WS, et al. Remote patient monitoring in chronic heart failure. Cardiology in Review. 2013;**21**:141-150

[30] McAlister FA, Stewart S, Ferrua S, et al. Multidisciplinary strategies for the management of heart failure patients at high risk for admission: A systematic review of randomized trials. Journal of the American College of Cardiology. 2004;**44**:810-819

[31] Riegel B, Moser DK, Anker SD, et al. State of the science: Promoting self-care in persons with heart failure: A scientific statement from the American Heart Association. Circulation. 2009;**120**:1141-1163

[32] Jaarsma T, Stromberg A, Ben Gal T, et al. Comparison of self-care behaviors of heart failure patients in 15 countries worldwide. Patient Education and Counseling. 2013;**92**:114-120

[33] Nieuwenhuis MM, Jaarsma T, van Veldhuisen DJ, et al. Factors associated with patient delay in seeking care after worsening symptoms in heart failure patients. Journal of Cardiac Failure. 2011;**17**:657-663

[34] Gallagher R, Luttik ML, Jaarsma T. Social support and self-care in heart failure. The Journal of Cardiovascular Nursing. 2011;**26**:439-445

Chapter 4

Critical Care of Acute Heart Failure

Chih-Hsin Hsu and Wei-Ting Li

Additional information is available at the end of the chapter

http://dx.doi.org/10.5772/intechopen.81721

Abstract

Acute heart failure is a life-threatening medical condition. Improving acute heart failure care is important. Early diagnosis and evaluating the etiology are important in acute heart failure. Patients with suspected acute heart failure should have a diagnostic workup, and appropriate pharmacological and nonpharmacological management should be started promptly and in parallel. Diagnosis of acute heart failure should be based on history and symptoms. The physical examination typically presents with some combination of increased congestion and decreased peripheral perfusion, further confirmed by electrocardiogram, chest radiograph, biomarkers, and echocardiogram. The first step in the management of a patient is to address life-threatening issues. Patients with respiratory failure or cardiogenic shock should be treated soon. The next step is the identification of precipitants that needs urgent management. Evidence-based medication to reduce morbidity and mortality for patients with heart failure includes an angiotensin converting enzyme inhibitor, angiotensin receptor blocker, or angiotensin receptor-neprilysin inhibitor; a beta blocker; and a mineralocorticoid receptor antagonist. During an acute heart failure episode, management of these agents depends upon whether the patient has contraindications to therapy such as hemodynamic instability or acute kidney injury. Once the patient is stable, therapies are carefully initiated, reinitiated, or titrated with appropriate follow-up.

Keywords: acute heart failure, critical care

1. Introduction

Acute heart failure is a relevant public health problem causing a majority of hospital admissions in patients aged of 65 years or more. Despite major achievements in the treatment of chronic heart failure over the last decades, which led to marked improvement in long-term survival, outcomes of acute heart failure remain poor with 90-day rehospitalization and 1-year mortality rates reaching 10–30%. There is an unmet need for improving acute heart failure care, including critical care to patient's outcome.

2. Critical care of acute heart failure

2.1. Introduction

Acute heart failure (AHF) is a disease with high rehospitalization and mortality rates. Improving acute heart failure critical care is important.

2.2. Definition of acute heart failure

Acute heart failure (AHF), also known as acute decompensated heart failure or cardiac failure, refers to rapid onset or worsening of symptoms and/or signs of heart failure (HF). It is a life-threatening medical problem requiring evaluation and management soon.

AHF may present as a first occurrence or as a consequence of acute decompensation of chronic HF. AHF may be caused by primary cardiac dysfunction or precipitated by extrinsic factors, often in patients with chronic HF.

2.3. Management of acute heart failure

AHF is a life-threatening medical problem; thus, rapid transfer to the nearest hospital is essential, which has a cardiology department and coronary care/intensive care unit (CCU/ICU). Early diagnosis and evaluating the etiology are important in AHF. Therefore, all patients with suspected AHF should have a diagnostic workup and appropriate pharmacological and nonpharmacological management should be started promptly and in parallel.

2.4. Causes/precipitant factors

The most frequent primary causes of AHF include ischemic, inflammatory, arrhythmia, and acute valve insufficiency. Decompensation of chronic HF can occur without known precipitant factors, but more often with one or more factors, such as infection, uncontrolled hypertension, rhythm disturbances, or nonadherence with drugs/diet (**Table 1**) [1]. Some of them leading to decompensation, which need to be treated/corrected urgently, include acute coronary syndromes (ACS), hypertensive emergency, severe arrhythmias, acute mechanical cause underlying AHF, or acute pulmonary embolism [1].

2.5. Diagnosis

Initial diagnosis of AHF should be based on a thorough history assessing symptoms, prior cardiovascular history, and potential cardiac and noncardiac precipitants. The physical examination of a patient with AHF typically presents with some combination of increased congestion and, less frequently, decreased peripheral perfusion, further confirmed by appropriate additional investigations such as image and laboratory assessment (with specific biomarkers).

http://dx.doi.org/10.5772/intechopen.81721

Acute coronary syndrome
Arrhythmia (tachyarrhythmia and bradyarrhythmia)
Excessive rise in blood pressure
Nonadherence with diet intake or medications
Toxic substances (alcohol, recreational drugs)
Drugs (e.g., NSAID, corticosteroid, cardiotoxic chemotherapeutics)
Exacerbation of chronic obstruction pulmonary disease
Pulmonary embolism
Surgery
Stress
Metabolic/hormonal derangements
Cerebrovascular insult
Acute mechanical cause

Table 1. Factors triggering acute heart failure.

2.5.1. *The information from physical examination*

2.5.1.1. *Vital sign*

Poorly controlled hypertension is one of the predictor factors of AHF and should be avoided. Hypotension is a dangerous sign of poor prognosis for patients with AHF. Unstable heart rate and rhythm are not only a cause of the AHF episode, but also increase the risk of unstable hemodynamic. Respiratory rate is often not as carefully assessed clinically as other vital signs, but may represent inadequate resolution of the initial episode of lung edema or a new event, such as a pulmonary embolus. Fever reflects the possibility of underlying infectious process, which can instigate AHF exacerbations. Oxygen saturation is also an important vital sign for HF patients and should be measured.

2.5.1.2. *Body weight*

Body weight provides an important information of severity of fluid overload and response to therapy. It is easy to measure and should be obtained as early as possible. Urine output and daily input and output measures are provided in more detail, but many clinical practices appear to be more difficult.

2.5.1.3. *Jugular venous pressure*

Jugular venous pressure (JVP) is a useful physical examination finding to monitor fluid status and response to therapy in the AHF patient. Elevation of the JVP suggests that there is persistent volume overload and need more diuresis. JVP will be influenced by significant tricuspid regurgitation, while the elicitation of hepatojugular reflux can augment the interpretation.

2.5.1.4. Heart sound

Cardiac auscultation is very basic and an important skill to follow the presence and severity of extra heart sounds (S3 and S4) and murmurs. The appearance of an S3 is associated with elevated ventricular pressure and poor left ventricular function. The reduction in the intensity of mitral and tricuspid regurgitation murmurs are the sign of reduction of ventricular filling pressure and volume.

2.5.1.5. Breath sound

Breath sound examination can provide the signs of lung congestion or pleural effusion. It can also evaluate the possibility of an underlying pneumonia.

2.5.1.6. Extremities

Extremities edema reflects the status of fluid overload, and extremities temperature reflects the distal perfusion. Both of them should be closely monitored to understand the severity of low cardiac output/fluid overload and the response to management.

2.5.2. What biochemistry studies should be ordered to help establish the diagnosis?

B-type natriuretic peptide (BNP) and N-terminal-proBNP BNP (NT-proBNP)—plasma concentrations of BNP and NT-proBNP—are increased in the presence of elevated ventricular pressure and volume, and have been used to assist in the diagnosis of AHF. There is no absolute "diagnostic level" of these biomarkers for AHF; most use different ranges. For example, a BNP less than or equal to 100 pg/mL is strongly suggestive of nonheart failure etiology for the dyspnea, BNP greater than 400 pg/mL is strongly supportive of AHF and BNP 100–400 pg/mL is indeterminate. High BNP levels may be the result of factors other than HF (e.g., age, renal dysfunction, myocardial infarction, acute pulmonary embolism, and high output states such as cirrhosis), and some factors may cause lower BNP levels (e.g., obesity, within 1 hour of flash pulmonary edema, acute mitral regurgitation, and mitral stenosis) [2–6].

Renal function markers: blood urea nitrogen (BUN) and creatinine are markers of renal function. Chronic renal insufficiency is a frequent comorbidity in patients with heart failure, and AHF episodes are often accompanied by acute on chronic renal failure.

Troponin: increased troponins reflect myocardial damage. ACS may precipitate AHF, but much more frequently, myocardium damage from AHF itself leading to mild-to-moderate troponin elevations. Distinguishing the "troponinemia" of heart failure from that of ACS or myocardial infarction can often be challenging and requires synthesis of symptoms and other clinical information [7].

2.5.3. What imaging studies should be ordered to help establish the diagnosis?

Electrocardiogram (ECG): the ECG can provide information of myocardial ischemia, chamber dilatation or hypertrophy, arrhythmias, and electrolyte disorders as contributing factors to AHF.

Chest radiography: the chest X-ray (CXR) can reflect pulmonary congestion or pleural effusions. Changes in cardiac silhouette may reflect cardiomegaly or pericardial effusion.

Echocardiogram: echocardiography is probably the most useful noninvasive imaging study for HF. It provides information on structure, and function of all cardiac chambers and valves. Potential wall motion abnormalities and estimates of hemodynamics were also able to be detected by echocardiography.

Pulmonary artery catheterization: the pulmonary artery (PA) catheter is a very useful diagnostic tool in properly selected patients. In patients with evidence of shock with unclear etiology, measurement of pulmonary capillary wedge pressures (PCWP), cardiac output, and vascular resistances can provide key information to guide appropriate selection of therapy. A PA catheter should not be routinely used in most patients with AHF due to potential complication (e.g., infection, vascular injury, etc.).

2.6. Clinical classification

Clinical classification can be based on physical examination to detect the presence of congestion ("wet" vs. "dry" if present vs. absent) and/or peripheral hypoperfusion ("cold" vs. "warm" if present vs. absent) [8, 9]. The combination of these options identifies four groups: warm and wet (well perfused and congested), cold and wet (hypoperfused and congested), cold and dry (hypoperfused without congestion), and warm and dry (compensated, well perfused without congestion). This classification may be helpful to guide therapy in the initial phase and carries prognostic information. The "cold and wet" groups have most poor prognosis and need urgent management [1, 8, 9] (**Figure 1**).

2.7. Monitor

2.7.1. Invasive monitor

The insertion of an arterial line in patients with AHF and cardiogenic shock was recommended. The arterial line allows for repetitive sampling of arterial blood gases, providing important information on oxygenation (PaO_2), ventilation ($PaCO_2$), acid-base balance, electrolytes, and lactate levels. The continuous measurement of arterial pressure allows for the appropriate titration of vasoactive medication.

The central venous catheter enables the monitoring of central venous pressure and allows the safe and continuous administration of vasoactive drugs and inotropes in patients with AHF who require intensive treatment. Central venous oxygen saturation ($ScvO_2$) can also be monitored with the central venous catheter. In combination with increased lactate levels and signs of organ dysfunction, $ScvO_2 < 60\%$ indicates severe hypoperfusion and mandates further diagnostics and urgent treatment.

A pulmonary artery catheter (PAC) may be considered in patients with hypotension and hypoperfusion to evaluate the volume status and cardiac output. However, the use of a PAC did not improve the survival and was associated with more adverse events. Based on the imbalance between potential benefits and known risks, PAC should not routinely be used to

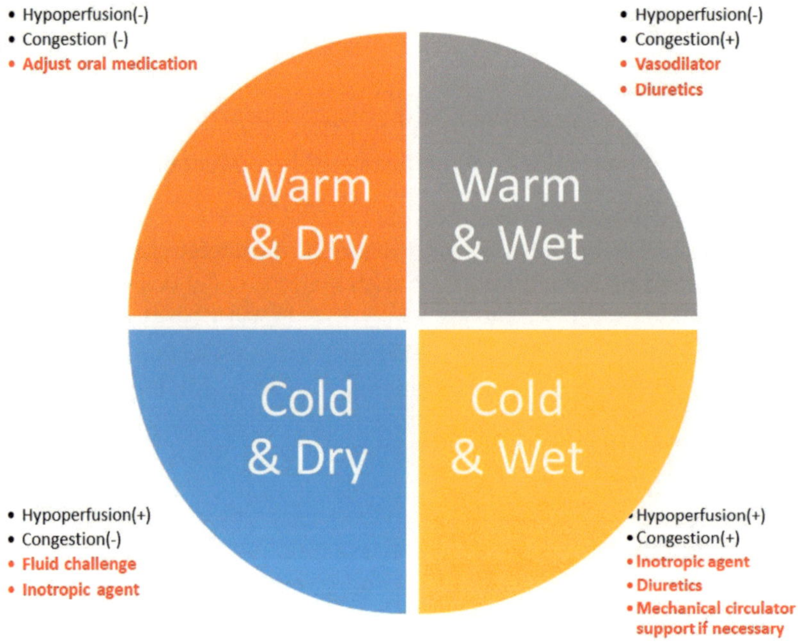

Figure 1. Classification and management of AHF.

monitor patients with AHF, but it can still be justified to use PAC in selected populations by experienced physicians. PAC is most appropriately used in critical patients who need rapid evaluation of vasoactive medications or fluid balance.

2.7.2. Noninvasive hemodynamic monitor

Noninvasive techniques are undergoing considerable development to avoid complications of invasive monitor. However, none can be currently recommended for routine clinical use. Invasive techniques such as the PAC and transpulmonary thermodilution remain the reference standard.

2.7.2.1. Contour of the pulse wave

Several algorithms have been proposed to determine cardiac output based on determination of systolic area by analysis of the contour of the pulse wave. These signals are often obtained from an arterial line.

2.7.2.2. Digital photoplethysmography

Digital photoplethysmography is a technique for continuous measurement of blood volume changes. Severe skin vasoconstriction, which is common in cardiogenic shock, impairs signal quality of blood pressure and is an important limitation of the technique. These monitors are not useful when arterial impedance is variable, such as with vasoconstrictor administration, unless given continuously and steady state has been reached. Digital photoplethysmography techniques do not appear to be sufficiently effective in assessing cardiac output in resuscitation patients with microcirculatory disorders, peripheral vasoconstriction, or high blood pressure lability.

2.7.2.3. *Thoracic bioimpedance*

Transthoracic electric bioimpedance is a noninvasive method for cardiac output measurement. Several hemodynamic parameters can be measured and calculated using the technique including flow (e.g., stroke volume/stroke index), resistance (e.g., systemic vascular resistance/index), contractility (e.g., cardiac power index, systolic time ratio, pre-ejection period, left ventricular ejection time, velocity index, acceleration index), and fluid (e.g., thoracic fluid content). Thoracic bioimpedance data may be useful in fluid management in patients with AHF, and the differentiation of cardiogenic from pulmonary causes of acute dyspnea. Bioimpedance might be useful for trend analysis, but the data should be interpreted cautiously, as the method is associated with limitations that may affect its accuracy (e.g., arrhythmias, mechanical ventilation, body motion, and factors that affect conductivity between the electrodes and the skin-like temperature and humidity).

2.8. Management

2.8.1. *First step*

The first step in management of the patient with AHF is to address life-threatening issues. Patients with respiratory distress/failure or cardiogenic shock should be treated soon and be triaged to a location where immediate respiratory and cardiovascular support can be provided.

2.8.1.1. *Respiratory failure*

Respiratory failure is the most frequent life-threatening condition for patients with AHF. Immediate management includes oxygen supply and removal of overload fluid.
Oxygen supply and ventilator support: immediate administration of supplemental oxygen is the most readily available means to improve oxygenation. If remain inadequate, rapid use of noninvasive ventilatory support continuous positive airway pressure or nasal intermittent positive pressure ventilation has been shown to be very effective in rapidly improving symptoms, hemodynamics, and metabolic abnormalities associated with AHF [10–12]. If noninvasive measures are insufficient, rapid intubation with mechanical positive pressure ventilation should be done.

Diuretic: most patients also have significant volume overload leading to the respiratory insufficiency, and diuretics remain the most commonly administered agent for AHF. Rapid administration of intravenous loop diuretics is recommended for volume overload and can relief symptoms quickly as well as decrease the underlying volume overload [13–15].

Ultrafiltration: potential benefits of ultrafiltration over intravenous diuretics include more effective removal of sodium, minimal effects on serum electrolytes, decreased neurohormonal activation, and adjustable and potentially very rapid fluid removal rates. The cost, need for vascular access, need for nursing training, and support are all potential barriers to ultrafiltration in clinical practice. Identifying the most appropriate patients for ultrafiltration therapy is an area of controversy and active clinical research.

2.8.1.2. Cardiogenic shock

Cardiogenic shock is defined as a hypotension (SBP < 90 mmHg) with signs of hypoperfusion (cold sweated extremities, oliguria, mental confusion, dizziness, narrow pulse pressure, etc.). Emergency management is necessary to improve organ perfusion by increasing cardiac output and blood pressure. After fluid challenge, pharmacologic management consists of positive inotropic agent and a vasopressor as needed. Positive inotropes agents and vasopressors used to treat acute heart failure are discussed below and listed in **Table 2**. However, rather than combining several inotropes, device therapy has to be considered when there is an inadequate response.

Positive inotropes: Positive inotropes increase heart contractility and cardiac output by increasing cAMP and intracellular calcium. Dobutamine is a predominant beta-1 adrenergic receptor agonist, which produces positive inotropic and chronotropic effects. The mechanism of action is the binding of the beta-1 receptor, leading to enhanced myocardial contractility. There is also a modest alpha and beta-2 effect, which causes mild peripheral vasodilation; in the context of increasing cardiac output, this can cause a variable effect on mean arterial pressure. The major side effects of dobutamine are atrial and ventricular tachyarrhythmias. Registry data of AHF patients suggest worse outcomes with dobutamine, and hence, its use is limited to patients with poor response to diuretics and vasodilators and patients in overt cardiogenic shock [16, 17]. Dopamine has variable effects on different receptors at different doses; conventionally at low doses (0–2 mcg/kg/min), there is preferential dopamine receptor activation leading to enhanced renal artery vasodilation and enhanced renal perfusion; at 2–10 mcg/kg/min, there is enhanced norepinephrine release, leading to enhanced myocardial contractility and mild peripheral vasoconstriction; at doses above 10 mcg/kg/min, there is preferential alpha adrenergic receptor activation causing peripheral vasoconstriction and an increase in mean arterial pressure [18]. Phosphodiesterase type III inhibitors, such as milrinone and enoximone, are a positive inotropic agent as well as a vasodilator. Its mechanism of action is the inhibition of the breakdown of cyclic adenosine monophosphate (cAMP) in cardiac myocytes, leading to the increase of cAMP-mediated Ca^{++} in the myocyte and hence enhanced myocyte contractility. Similarly, in the vascular smooth muscle, its action is that of increasing cAMP-mediated contractile protein phosphorylation, leading to vascular relaxation. The hemodynamic changes seen with milrinone include an increased cardiac output, decreased systemic vascular resistance, reduced PCWP, and typically a mild decrease in mean arterial pressure. Milrinone did not significantly decrease hospitalization length of stay, and did lead to significantly more hypotension and atrial arrhythmias. Increased myocardial ischemia and increased mortality in patients with ischemic heart disease may also occur. Although bolus loading was suggested, some clinicians no longer use a bolus loading dose to avoid significant hypotension. Patients should be carefully monitored in intensive care unit when used with milrinone [19–21]. Levosimendan is an ATP-dependent potassium channel activator with myocardial calcium sensitizing and possible PDE III inhibitor effects, and acts

http://dx.doi.org/10.5772/intechopen.81721

Inotropes/vasopressors	Dose	Recommended
Dobutamine (beta-1 adrenergic receptor agonist)	2–20 μg/kg/min	Also a vasodilator, may increase the risk of arrhythmia and hypotension
Dopamine (variable effects on different receptors at different dose)	3–5 μg/kg/min; inotropic (beta+) >5 μg/kg/min: (beta+), vasopressor (alpha+)	May increase the risk of arrhythmia
Milrinone (phosphodiesterase type III inhibitors)	25–75 μg/kg over 10–20 min (optional) 0.375–0.75 μg/kg/min	Also a vasodilator not recommended in acutely worsened ischemic heart failure. Dose adjustment is required in the presence of renal insufficiency, hypotension, or arrhythmias.
Enoximone (phosphodiesterase type III inhibitors)	0.5–1.0 mg/kg over 5–10 min (optional) 5–20 μg/kg/min	Also a vasodilator similar as Milrinone
Levosimendan (ATP-dependent potassium channel activator with myocardial calcium sensitizing effects and possible PDE III inhibitor effects)	12 μg/kg over 10 min (optional) 0.1 μg/kg/min, which can be decreased to 0.05 or increased to 0.2 μg/kg/min	Also a vasodilator increases the risk of hypotension
Norepinephrine (alpha agonist)	0.2–1.0 μg/kg/min	Increase systemic vascular resistance and afterload
Epinephrine (alpha and beta agonist)	0.05–0.5 μg/kg/min	Increase the risk of arrhythmia

Table 2. Positive inotropes and/or vasopressors for acute heart failure.

as a vasodilator and inotrope. Hypotension and arrhythmias may occur, and patients should be carefully monitored. Using a bolus loading dose or not depends on the blood pressure [22–24]. Monitoring of response to these therapies depends upon the hemodynamic, peripheral perfusion, and other target organ functions.

Vasopressors: Drugs with peripheral arterial vasoconstrictor action such as norepinephrine or dopamine in higher doses (5 mg/kg/min) are given to patients with marked hypotension. These agents are given to raise blood pressure and redistribute blood to the vital organs. However, LV afterload increases under vasopressors use. A subgroup analysis suggested that norepinephrine would have fewer side effects and lower mortality [25]. Epinephrine (adrenaline) should be restricted to patients with persistent hypotension despite adequate cardiac filling pressures and the use of other vasoactive agents, as well as for resuscitation protocols [26].

Mechanical circulatory support: In cases of severe AHF, which is refractory to medical therapy, temporary circulatory support (TCS) can be utilized to improve end organ perfusion. TCS ranges from percutaneously inserted devices, such as intra-aortic balloon pump (IABP) to ventricular assist devices (VAD). IABP can be used at many centers for severe cardiac compromise and provide benefits in decreasing afterload and increasing coronary infusion and cardiac output. The contraindication is moderate-to-severe aortic insufficiency and aortic aneurysms/dissections, and is limited by vascular access issues and complications. IABP could only partial increase cardiac output, and there is no benefit for right heart failure. In cases of complete hemodynamic collapse or severe right ventricular failure, other mechanical support devices may be used at specialized centers, including VADs and extracorporeal membrane oxygenation (ECMO). ECMO can be placed to completely bypass the cardiopulmonary circulation. Additional surgically placed TCS includes semidurable continuous-flow ventricular assist devices. TCS can serve as a "bridge to recovery" or as a "bridge to decision" in patients who may need implantation of permanent LV assist devices or cardiac transplantation.

2.8.2. Second step

The next step to identification of precipitants/causes leading to decompensation that needs urgent management, including ACS, hypertensive emergency, arrhythmia, acute mechanical cause underlying AHF, and pulmonary embolism [1].

Acute coronary syndrome: coexistence of ACS and AHF identifies a very-high-risk group where an immediate invasive strategy with intent to perform revascularization is recommended [27, 28].

Hypertensive emergency: aggressive blood pressure reduction (in the range of 25% during the first few hours and cautiously thereafter) should be considered and initiated as soon as possible with i.v. vasodilators in combination with loop diuretics, which is recommended [29, 30].

Arrhythmias: severe rhythm disturbances in patients with AHF and unstable conditions should be corrected urgently with medical therapy, electrical cardioversion, or temporary pacing [31, 32].

Acute mechanical cause underlying AHF: this may present as a complication of ACS (free wall rupture, ventricular septal defect, or acute mitral regurgitation), chest trauma or cardiac intervention, or as acute valve incompetence. Echocardiography is essential for diagnosis, and treatment typically requires emergency surgical repair. Surgery might not be performed soon in some special consideration. Patients suffer from postmyocardial infarction ventricular septal defect, and acute mitral regurgitation with acceptable hemodynamic might use IABP to unload ventricular pressure and perform surgery several days later till cardiac muscle inflammation improved.

Acute pulmonary embolism: patients presenting with acute pulmonary embolism should be managed according to the guidelines. Immediate reperfusion either with thrombolysis, catheter-based approach, or surgical embolectomy is recommended if hemodynamically unstable [33].

2.8.3. Other medications for AHF

2.8.3.1. Vasodilator therapy

Use of vasodilator therapy in patients with AHF is based upon hemodynamic response, since evidence on efficacy and safety of vasodilatory therapy in AHF is limited. The routine use of vasodilators does not improve outcomes, and should be avoided [30, 34, 35].

Nitrates: nitrates can be very effective as vasodilators, producing rapid decreases in pulmonary congestion, left ventricular end diastolic pressure, LV wall stress, and myocardial oxygen consumption. Rapid administration of intravenous nitrates in patients with severe pulmonary edema decreased the need for mechanical ventilation and myocardial infarction compared to a high-dose furosemide strategy in a randomized study. It has coronary vasodilatory effects as well, making it a good option for patient with ongoing ischemia. Initial intravenous dose is typically 20 mcg/min, with a doubling of the dose every 5–15 min. Other options for administration include sublingual tablets and sprays as well as topical pastes. Major side effects include hypotension and headache.

Nesiritide: nesiritide is a recombinant B-type natriuretic peptide. It has balanced venous and arteriolar actions, and modestly enhances diuresis through direct renal effects. The dose starts at 0.01 mcg/kg/min. Though there may be a role for nesiritide in some special populations (i.e., diuretic-resistant patients), however, there was a higher rate of hypotension and there was no significant change in the rate of death, rehospitalization, or renal function. Routine use of nesiritide in acute decompensate heart failure was not recommended.

2.8.3.2. Digoxin

Digoxin is mostly indicated in patients with AHF and rapid ventricular rate. However, in patients with renal failure or other factors affecting digoxin metabolism (including other drugs and elderly), the maintenance dose should be adjusted and avoid overdose.

2.8.4. Management of evidence-based oral therapies

Evidence-based medication to reduce morbidity and mortality for patients with chronic HF includes an angiotensin-converting enzyme (ACE) inhibitor, angiotensin receptor blocker (ARB), or angiotensin receptor-neprilysin inhibitor (ARNI); a beta blocker; and a mineralocorticoid receptor antagonist (MRA). During an acute HF episode, management of these agents depends upon whether the patient was already receiving these medications and whether the patient has contraindications to therapy such as hemodynamic instability or acute kidney injury. Once the patient is stable, evidence-based therapies are carefully initiated, reinitiated, or titrated with arrangements for appropriate outpatient follow-up. In stable patients, ACE inhibitor, ARB, or ARNI and beta blocker therapy should be initiated prior to hospital discharge, and then MRA should be added as soon as possible. Ivabradine reduces the risk of hospitalization in patients with HF and can increase stroke volume and maintain cardiac output when heart rate slows down. Ivabradine may be considered to be used with dobutamine at the acute phase [36, 37].

2.8.5. Common pitfalls and side effects of management

Management of patients with AHF is complex and highly specific to the individual. However, there are some common pitfalls:

Hypotension: most therapies for AHF can cause hypotension, and the development of hypotension related to poor clinical outcomes. Blood pressure, central venous pressure, body weight, urine output, and renal function should carefully be monitored to avoid hypotension. If hypotension happens, rapidly evaluate the perfusion and delete vasodilator (be especially aware of nitrates), and position the patient as necessary to improve perfusion. In many patients, raising the legs will provide sufficient augmentation of venous return to improve symptoms.

Worsening renal function: since worsening renal function can result from inadequate diuresis or be the result of excessive diuresis with volume depletion. In these situations, measurements of baseline BUN and creatinine as comparators and central venous pressure are very helpful to have treatment decision. Transient decreases in renal function may not portend the poor prognosis, as previously believed, and may just reflect the response to therapy.

Electrolyte imbalance: electrolyte imbalance is often noted under diuretic use and might lead to life-threatening arrhythmias. Close monitoring and positive correction are necessary.

3. Conclusion

- The first step in management of the patient with AHF is to address life-threatening issues. Patients with respiratory distress/failure or hemodynamic compromise should be treated soon.
- Respiratory failure should be treated first; initial therapy includes supplemental oxygen and assisted ventilation. Patients with respiratory failure due to AHF who fail to improve with non invasive ventilation require endotracheal intubation for conventional mechanical ventilation.
- Most patients will also have significant volume overload leading to the respiratory insufficiency; diuretics remain the most commonly administered agent for AHF. Rapid administration of intravenous loop diuretics is recommended for volume overload. Ultrafiltration should be performed if failed to improve under diuretics use.
- Severe low cardiac output requires aggressive management of their shock to mitigate or prevent the related end organ damage. Positive inotropes agents and vasopressors are used to treat low cardiac output and hypotension. In cases of severe AHF, which is refractory to medical therapy, temporary circulatory support (TCS) can be utilized to improve end-organ perfusion.
- The next step to identification of precipitants/causes leading to decompensation that needs urgent management, including acute coronary syndrome, hypertensive emergency, arrhythmia, and acute mechanical and pulmonary embolism.
- Vasodilators may be required to correct elevated filling pressures. The routine use of vasodilators does not improve outcomes, and should be avoided.
- Evidence-based medication to reduce morbidity and mortality for patients with chronic HF includes an angiotensin converting enzyme (ACE) inhibitor, angiotensin receptor blocker (ARB), or angiotensin receptor-neprilysin inhibitor (ARNI); a beta blocker; and a mineralocorticoid receptor antagonist (MRA). During an acute HF episode, management of these agents depends upon whether the patient was already receiving these medications and whether the patient has contraindications to therapy such as hemodynamic instability or acute kidney injury. Once the patient is stable, evidence-based therapies are carefully initiated.

Conflict of interest

None.

http://dx.doi.org/10.5772/intechopen.81721

Author details

Chih-Hsin Hsu* and Wei-Ting Li

*Address all correspondence to: chihhsinhsu@gmail.com

National Cheng Kung University Hospital, Tainan, Taiwan

References

[1] Ponikowski P, Voors AA, Anker SD, Bueno H, Cleland JGF, Coats AJS, et al. 2016 ESC guidelines for the diagnosis and treatment of acute and chronic heart failure. European Heart Journal. 2016;**37**:2129-2200

[2] Fuat A, Murphy JJ, Hungin APS, Curry J, Mehrzad AA, Hetherington A, et al. The diagnostic accuracy and utility of a B-type natriuretic peptide test in a community population of patients with suspected heart failure. The British Journal of General Practice. 2006;**56**:327-333

[3] Yamamoto K, Burnett JC, Bermudez EA, Jougasaki M, Bailey KR, Redfield MM. Clinical criteria and biochemical markers for the detection of systolic dysfunction. Journal of Cardiac Failure. 2000;**6**:194-200

[4] Cowie MR, Struthers AD, Wood DA, Coats AJ, Thompson SG, Poole-Wilson PA, et al. Value of natriuretic peptides in assessment of patients with possible new heart failure in primary care. Lancet. 1997;**350**:1349-1353

[5] Krishnaswamy P, Lubien E, Clopton P, Koon J, Kazanegra R, Wanner E, et al. Utility of B-natriuretic peptide levels in identifying patients with left ventricular systolic or diastolic dysfunction. The American Journal of Medicine. 2001;**111**:274-279

[6] Kelder JC, Cramer MJ, Verweij WM, Grobbee DE, Hoes AW. Clinical utility of three B-type natriuretic peptide assays for the initial diagnostic assessment of new slow-onset heart failure. Journal of Cardiac Failure. 2011;**17**:729-734

[7] Felker GM, Mentz RJ, Teerlink JR, Voors AA, Pang PS, Ponikowski P, et al. Serial high sensitivity cardiac troponin T measurement in acute heart failure: Insights from the RELAX-AHF study. European Journal of Heart Failure. 2015;**17**:1262-1270

[8] Nohria A, Tsang SW, Fang JC, Lewis EF, Jarcho JA, Mudge GH, et al. Clinical assessment identifies hemodynamic profiles that predict outcomes in patients admitted with heart failure. Journal of the American College of Cardiology. 2003;**41**:1797-1804

[9] Stevenson LW. Design of therapy for advanced heart failure. European Journal of Heart Failure. 2005;**7**:323-331

[10] Weng C-L, Zhao Y-T, Liu Q-H, Fu C-J, Sun F, Ma Y-L, et al. Meta-analysis: Noninvasive ventilation in acute cardiogenic pulmonary edema. Annals of Internal Medicine. 2010;**152**:590-600

[11] Park M, Sangean MC, Volpe MDS, Feltrim MIZ, Nozawa E, Leite PF, et al. Randomized, prospective trial of oxygen, continuous positive airway pressure, and bilevel positive airway pressure by face mask in acute cardiogenic pulmonary edema. Critical Care Medicine. 2004;**32**:2407-2415

[12] Gray A, Goodacre S, Newby DE, Masson M, Sampson F, Nicholl J, et al. Noninvasive ventilation in acute cardiogenic pulmonary edema. The New England Journal of Medicine. 2008;**359**:142-151

[13] Felker GM, O'Connor CM, Braunwald E. Heart Failure Clinical Research Network Investigators. Loop diuretics in acute decompensated heart failure: Necessary? Evil? A necessary evil? Circulation. Heart Failure. 2009;**2**:56

[14] Stampfer M, Epstein SE, Beiser GD, Braunwald E. Hemodynamic effects of diuresis at rest and during intense upright exercise in patients with impaired cardiac function. Circulation. 1968;**37**:900

[15] Matsue Y, Damman K, Voors AA, et al. Time-to-furosemide treatment and mortality in patients hospitalized with acute heart failure. Journal of the American College of Cardiology. 2017;**69**:3042

[16] Liang CS, Sherman LG, Doherty JU, et al. Sustained improvement of cardiac function in patients with congestive heart failure after short-term infusion of dobutamine. Circulation. 1984;**69**:113

[17] Unverferth DV, Magorien RD, Lewis RP, Leier CV. Long-term benefit of dobutamine in patients with congestive cardiomyopathy. American Heart Journal. 1980;**100**:622

[18] Elkayam U, Ng TM, Hatamizadeh P, et al. Renal vasodilatory action of dopamine in patients with heart failure: Magnitude of effect and site of action. Circulation. 2008;**117**:200

[19] Cuffe MS, Califf RM, Adams KF Jr, et al. Short-term intravenous milrinone for acute exacerbation of chronic heart failure: A randomized controlled trial. JAMA. 2002;**287**:1541

[20] Simonton CA, Chatterjee K, Cody RJ, et al. Milrinone in congestive heart failure: Acute and chronic hemodynamic and clinical evaluation. Journal of the American College of Cardiology. 1985;**6**:453

[21] Anderson JL. Hemodynamic and clinical benefits with intravenous milrinone in severe chronic heart failure: Results of a multicenter study in the United States. American Heart Journal. 1991;**121**:1956

[22] Mebazaa A, Nieminen MS, Filippatos GS, Cleland JG, Salon JE, Thakkar R, et al. Levosimendan vs. dobutamine: Outcomes for acute heart failure patients on b-blockers in SURVIVE. European Journal of Heart Failure. 2009;**11**:304-311

[23] Pathak A, Lebrin M, Vaccaro A, Senard JM, Despas F. Pharmacology of levosimendan: Inotropic, vasodilatory and cardioprotective effects. Journal of Clinical Pharmacy and Therapeutics. 2013;**38**:341-349

[24] Papp Z, Edes I, Fruhwald S, De Hert SG, Salmenpera M, Leppikangas H, et al. Levosimendan: Molecular mechanisms and clinical implications: Consensus of experts on the mechanisms of action of levosimendan. International Journal of Cardiology. 2012;**159**:82-87

[25] De Backer D, Biston P, Devriendt J, Madl C, Chochrad D, Aldecoa C, et al. Comparison of dopamine and norepinephrine in the treatment of shock. The New England Journal of Medicine. 2010;**362**:779-789

[26] Monsieurs KG, Nolan JP, Bossaert LL, Greif R, Maconochie IK, Nikolaou NI, et al. European resuscitation council guidelines for resuscitation 2015: Section 1. Executive summary. Resuscitation. 2015;**95**:1-80

[27] Roffi M, Patrono C, Collet J-P, Mueller C, Valgimigli M, Andreotti F, et al. 2015 ESC guidelines for the management of acute coronary syndromes in patients presenting without persistent ST-segment elevation. European Heart Journal. 2016;**37**(3):267-315 ehv320

[28] Task Force on the management of ST-segment elevation acute myocardial infarction of the European Society of Cardiology (ESC), Steg PG, James SK, Atar D, Badano LP, Blömstrom-Lundqvist C, et al. ESC guidelines for the management of acute myocardial infarction in patients presenting with ST-segment elevation. European Heart Journal. 2012;**33**:2569-2619

[29] Levy P, Compton S, Welch R, Delgado G, Jennett A, Penugonda N, et al. Treatment of severe decompensated heart failure with high-dose intravenous nitroglycerin: A feasibility and outcome analysis. Annals of Emergency Medicine. 2007;**50**:144-152

[30] Cotter G, Metzkor E, Kaluski E, Faigenberg Z, Miller R, Simovitz A, et al. Randomised trial of high-dose isosorbide dinitrate plus low-dose furosemide versus high-dose furosemide plus low-dose isosorbide dinitrate in severe pulmonary edema. Lancet. 1998;**351**:389-393

[31] Priori SG, Blomström-Lundqvist C, Mazzanti A, Blom N, Borggrefe M, Camm J, et al. 2015 ESC guidelines for the management of patients with ventricular arrhythmias and the prevention of sudden cardiac death: The task force for the management of patients with ventricular arrhythmias and the prevention of sudden cardiac death of the Europe. European Heart Journal. 2015;**36**:2793-2867

[32] Brignole M, Auricchio A, Baron-Esquivias G, Bordachar P, Boriani G, Breithardt O-A, et al. 2013 ESC guidelines on cardiac pacing and cardiac resynchronization therapy: The task force on cardiac pacing and resynchronization therapy of the European Society of Cardiology (ESC). Developed in collaboration with the European heart rhythm association. European Heart Journal. 2013;**34**:2281-2329

[33] Konstantinides SV, Torbicki A, Agnelli G, Danchin N, Fitzmaurice D, Galiè N, et al. 2014 ESC guidelines on the diagnosis and management of acute pulmonary embolism. European Heart Journal. 2014;**35**:3033-3073

[34] Sharon A, Shpirer I, Kaluski E, et al. High-dose intravenous isosorbide-dinitrate is safer and better than Bi-PAP ventilation combined with conventional treatment for severe pulmonary edema. Journal of the American College of Cardiology. 2000;**36**:832

[35] O'Connor CM, Starling RC, Hernandez AF, et al. Effect of nesiritide in patients with acute decompensated heart failure. The New England Journal of Medicine. 2011;**365**:32

[36] Bakkehaug JP, Naesheim T, Torgersen Engstad E, Kildal AB, Myrmel T, How OJ. Reversing dobutamine-induced tachycardia using ivabradine increases stroke volume with neutral effect on cardiac energetics in left ventricular post-ischaemia dysfunction. Acta Physiologica. 2016;**218**(2):78-88

[37] Gallet R, Ternacle J, Damy T, Guendouz S, Bremont C, Seemann A, et al. Hemodynamic effects of Ivabradine in addition to dobutamine in patients with severe systolic dysfunction. International Journal of Cardiology. 2014;**176**:450-455

Chapter 5

Heart Failure in Sub-Saharan Africa

Okechukwu S. Ogah, Adewole Adebiyi and
Karen Sliwa

Additional information is available at the end of the chapter

http://dx.doi.org/10.5772/intechopen.82416

Abstract

Sub-Saharan Africa (SSA) is currently experiencing multiple burden of disease as a result of demographic and epidemiologic transition. This is occasioned rapid urbanization, unhealthy diets rich in fats and salt, western lifestyle and sedentary living. Heart failure (HF) has become a global public health issue. It is associated with high morbidity and mortality, frequent hospitalization and high economic cost. In SSA, HF is a disease of young and middle-aged adults with the attendant high disability-adjusted life years. This is unlike to the clinical profile and pattern of HF in high-income countries of North America, Western Europe and Japan where HF is a disease of the elderly. In addition, while ischaemic heart disease is the commonest aetiologic risk factor for HF in high income countries, HF in SSA is essentially non-ischaemic in origin. Hypertensive heart failure, dilated cardiomyopathy, rheumatic heart disease, pericardial diseases and HIV associated cardiomyopathy are the common risk factors. The chapter reviews the contemporary information on HF in SSA in terms of socio-demographic features, clinical characteristics, aetiological risk factors, management, prognosis and economic burden.

Keywords: heart failure, cardiac failure, cardiac dysfunction, sub-Saharan Africa, Africa

1. Introduction

Africa has multiple burden of disease. While the continent is still grabbling with traditional communicable and infectious diseases, there is increasing burden of non-communicable diseases (NCDs) such as hypertension, diabetes mellitus, cancers, etc., in addition to HIV/AIDS, malnutrition, wars and conflicts. The rapid epidemiologic transition from communicable to non-communicable diseases can be attributed to rapid urbanization, unhealthy diets rich in fats and salt, western lifestyle and sedentary living.

The global burden of disease 2015 report ranked NCDs only second to HIV/AIDS as the commonest cause of morbidity and mortality in SSA. It is projected that in the near future, NCDs will become the bigger cause of mortality in the region.

Like in other parts of the world, heart failure (HF) is associated with high morbidity and mortality, frequent hospitalization and high economic cost. In sub-Saharan Africa, HF has been shown to affect young and middle-aged adults with the attendant high disability-adjusted life years. This is contrary to the pattern of HF in high-income countries of North America, Western Europe and Japan where HF is essentially a disease of the elderly. Furthermore, while ischaemic heart disease is the commonest aetiologic risk factor for HF in high-income countries, HF in SSA is essentially non-ischaemic in origin. Hypertensive heart failure, dilated cardiomyopathy, rheumatic heart disease, pericardial diseases and HIV-associated cardiomyopathy are the common risk factors.

The aim of this chapter is to review contemporary information on HF in SSA in terms of sociodemographic features, clinical characteristics, aetiological risk factors, management, prognosis and economic burden. We shall conclude with gaps in knowledge and possible feature directions.

2. Sub-Saharan Africa

SSA is the geographical term used to describe the region of the African continent that lies south of the Sahara Desert. It covers a land area of 24.3 million square meters. In 2007, the

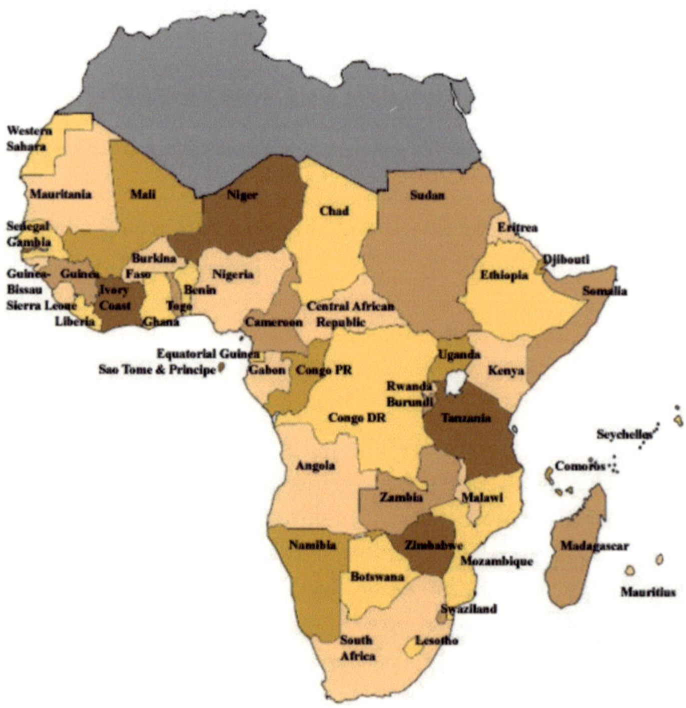

Figure 1. Map of sub-Saharan Africa.

http://dx.doi.org/10.5772/intechopen.82416

population of the region was estimated to 800 million with a growth rate of 2.3% per annum. The United Nation has projected a population of 1.5 billion by 2050 [1]. **Figure 1** shows the countries that comprise the region including the sub-regions of: (1) West Africa, (2) Central Africa or Middle Africa, (3) Eastern Africa, (4) Horn of Africa and (5) Southern Africa. [2] The population of SSA is very diverse both physically and culturally and they have differing ethnic background. For instance, the Negroes inhabit most of West Africa; the Tuaregs Nilo-Hamites occupy the east horn of the continent, while the Bantus inhabit the Central and Southern Africa. There are also the Hottentots in rural Namibia and the pygmies of the Congo Basin [2].

3. Historical perspective

Albert Ruskin Cooke [3] appears to be one of the earliest workers to have reported on the pattern of diseases in Africa. In 1901, he analysed 1500 in-patients, whom he met at a hospital in Uganda. He observed that 3% of all hospital admissions and 6% of all medical admissions were due to heart disease. He wrote 'Valvular diseases of the heart are common', 'Atheroma and aneurysms are very rare, although syphilitic endarteritis obliterans is probably common' and 'high tension pulses are not often met with' [4].

Fifty years later, Sharper and his colleagues analysed 1957 medical admission seen at the Mulago Hospital in Kampala and noted that cardiovascular disease was responsible for 8–10% of medical admissions. The main cardiac conditions reported were hypertensive heart disease, rheumatic heart disease, endomyocardial fibrosis and syphilitic heart disease [5, 6].

Similar work carried out in other countries in the 1960s and 1970s reported similar percentage that cardiovascular diseases are of all medical admissions. For example, 11.2% for Ibadan, Nigeria [7], 8.6% for Mombasa, Kenya [8], 8.8% for Dar es Salaam, Tanzania [9], 4.3% for Blantyre, Malawi [10] and 8.6% for Sekhukhuneland, South Africa [11].

Studies in the late 1970s, 1980s and in the 1990s also show the prominence of hypertensive heart disease, rheumatic heart disease and dilated cardiomyopathy as the main causes of heart disease in the region and decreasing incidence of syphilitic heart disease.

More recent studies have used echocardiography in the evaluation of heart diseases in the region. These have documented peculiar characteristics of heart diseases in sub-Saharan Africa [12–20].

4. Contemporary epidemiology of HF in SSA

4.1. Incidence and prevalence

There is lack of population-based incidence and prevalence studies in SSA. The reported hospital prevalence studies indicate that HF is responsible for 9.4–42.5% of all medical admissions and 25.6–30.0% of admissions into the cardiac units.

4.2. Socio-demographic characteristics

4.2.1. Age at presentation

HF in SSA is a disease of young and middle age. It is commoner between the third and fifth decade of life when the individuals are in the prime of their life. The mean age ranges from 36.5 to 61.5 years (**Figure 2A**) [15, 19–33]. In high-income countries, it is commoner in the seventh decade of life.

4.2.2. Gender distribution

There is varying gender distribution. It is commoner in men in countries where hypertensive heart disease is the commonest aetiology. Women are predominating where rheumatic heart disease and cardiomyopathies (peripartum cardiomyopathy) is common (**Figure 2B**) [15, 18–39].

4.3. Clinical profile

4.3.1. Mode of presentation and diagnosis

Most patients present in advanced heart failure (NYHA class III and IV) [26, 40]. Diagnosis of HF in SSA is mostly based on clinical features, mostly by the Framingham criteria (in 28.6%)

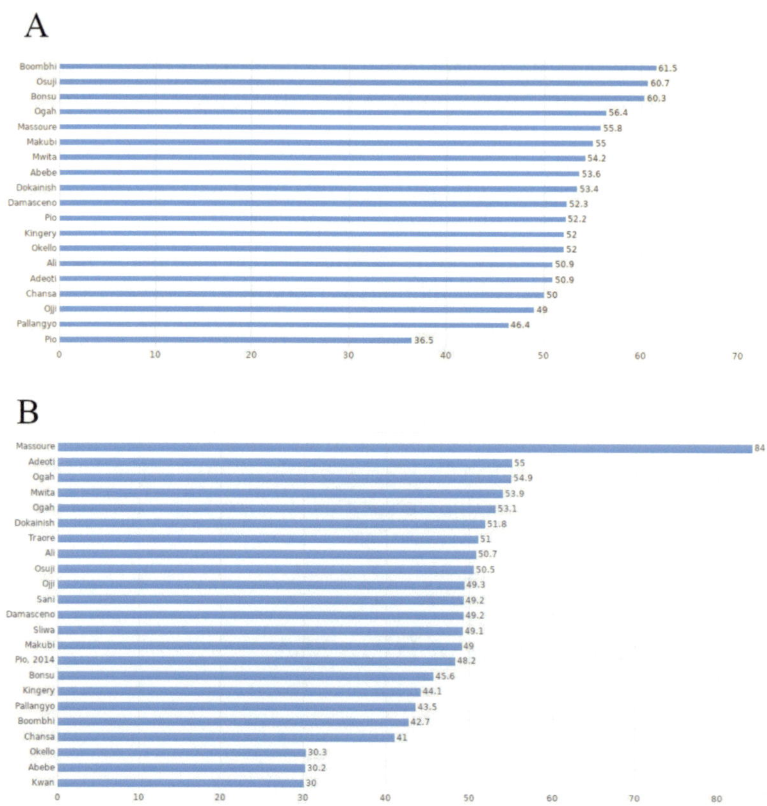

Figure 2. (A) Mean age of HF patients from various studies in SSA. (B) Proportion of men in various HF studies in SSA.

and European Society of Cardiology criteria (in 20%). Support facilities and services for diagnosis of HF in SSA are generally lacking in many parts of SSA [41]. Common diagnostic tools employed are chest radiography, 12-lead ECG and echocardiography. Biomarkers are less often used because of non-availability and high cost [39, 42].

4.3.2. Symptoms and signs

Common symptoms of HF in SSA include cough, dyspnoea, orthopnoea, paroxysmal nocturnal dyspnoea, pedal oedema and easy fatiguability. Rales, displaced apex beat, elevated jugular venous pressure and third heart sound are common signs. Others include peripheral oedema, tender hepatomegaly and systolic murmur [18].

Baseline rales and change to day 7 or discharge in general well-being are associated with death or readmission through 180 days. In addition, baseline orthopnoea, rales, oedema, oxygen saturation and changes to day 7 or discharge in respiratory rate or general well-being have been shown to be predictive of 6-months readmission or death [37].

4.3.3. Clinical class of heart failure

HF patients in SSA most often than not present in severe HF (NYHA class III and IV) [26, 27, 40].

In the INTER-CHF study, 35.5 and 20.9% of African HF patients were in NYHA classes III and IV, respectively.

4.3.4. Precipitating factors

Precipitants of HF in SSA are infections (especially chest and urinary tract infection), uncontrolled hypertension and arrhythmias especially atrial fibrillation. Other precipitants include anaemia, excessive physical activity and electrolyte imbalance (e.g. hyponatremia and hypokalemia) [17, 18, 43].

5. Aetiology HF in SSA

Hypertensive heart disease is the identified number one risk factor for HF in SSA. It is responsible for about 39.2% (95% CI: 32.6–45.9%). This is followed by dilated cardiomyopathy, 22.7% (95% CI: 16.8–29.1%) and rheumatic heart disease, 13.8% (95% CI: 9.9–18.0%). These three aetiological risk factors are responsible for over 75% of HF in the region. Ischaemic heart disease accounts for about 7.2% (95% CI: 4.1–11%). The general trend is that ischaemic heart disease is gradually rising in many parts of SSA. **Table 1** shows the aetiology of HF from recent publications from SSA.

5.1. Aetiological risk factor for HF in SSA

5.1.1. Hypertensive heart disease

Many years ago, Donnison [44] reported that hypertension was uncommon in Africa. This observation was later supported by the post-mortem studies by workers like Jex-Blake [45],

Author	Year	Country	Mode	Number	HHD (%)	DCM (%)	RHD (%)	IHD (%)	PPCM (%)	PDX	CHD(%)	CP (%)
Kingery [29]	2017	Tanzania	Prospective	145	42.8	19.3		6.2				7.6
Boombhi [21]	2017	Cameroon	Retrospective	148	30.16	28.57		6.35	3.18	3.96		8.73
Traore [35]	2017	Ivory Coast	Retrospective	257	22.9	55.57		11.23				
Ansa [209]	2016	Nigeria	Retrospective	144	48.6	35.4	1.4					
Abebe [25]	2016	Ethiopia	Retrospective	311	16.1	12.5		15.8				4.5
Dokainish [26]	2015	Multi-country	Prospective	1294	35	14.5	7.2	20				
Makubi [210]	2014	Tanzania	Prospective	427	45	28	12	9				
Ogah [18]	2014	Nigeria	Prospective	452	78.5	7.5	2.4	0.4		3.3		4.4
Pio [28]	2014	Togo	Prospective	297	43.1			19.2	11.8		2.7	2.7
Pio [32]	2014	Togo	Retrospective	376	42.8	5.8		2.7	15.4	1.1	2.7	2.1
Kwan [211]	2013	Rwanda	Retrospective	138	8	54	25	0				
Massoure [211]	2013	Djibouti	Prospective	45	18	7	13					
Ojji [212]	2013	Nigeria	Prospective	1515	60.6	12	8.6	0.4	5.3			
Damasceno [27]	2012	Multi-country	Prospective	1006	45.4	18.8	14.3	7.7	7.7	6.8		
Onwuchekwa [213]	2009	Nigeria	Retrospective	423	56.3	12.2	4.26	0.24			0.24	2.13
Stewart [17]	2008	South Africa	Prospective	884	33	35		9				
Ogah [34]	2008	Nigeria	Retrospective	1441	56.7	3	3.7	0.6		1.8		1.6
Familoni [214]	2007	Nigeria	Prospective	82	43.4	28	9.8	8.5				3.7
Owusu [215]	2007	Ghana	Prospective	167	42.5	17.4	21.6	3.6		4.2	2.4	2.4
Kingue [216]	2005	Cameroon	Retrospective	167	54.5	26.3	24.6	2.4				
Thiam [217]	2003	Senegal	Prospective	170	34			18.9				

HHD = hypertensive heart disease, DCM = dilated cardiomyopathy, RHD = rheumatic heart disease, IHD = ischaemic heart disease, PPCM = peripartum cardiomyopathy, CHD = congenital heart disease, PDX = pericardial disease, CP = cor pulmonale.

Table 1. Aetiology of heart failure in some studies conducted in SSA since the year 2000.

Vint [46] as well as clinical study by William [47] in 1941. However, by 1946, workers started reporting on the impact of hypertension on the cardiovascular health of the African. Davies [48] noted that hypertensive heart disease was the commonest cause of congestive heart failure in Kampala. Similar report was also noted in South Africa [49]. Within same period, many other authors from different parts of Africa also documented that the disease is common in the continent, occasionally with prevalence similar to data from Europe and America.

It is known that in isolated and primitive areas of the continent, the prevalence of hypertension is very low and in these populations, blood pressure remains within a narrow range throughout adult life [50]. Blood pressure rises modestly with age in rural dwellers and much more in those who live in the cities.

More recent data from the continent suggest that hypertension is a major cause of cardiac morbidity and mortality [51, 52]. High blood pressure is in fact regarded as the foundation of cardiovascular disease in Africa [53]. In a recent systematic review of hypertension survey in Africa, it was shown that hypertension increased from 54.6 million cases in 1990 to 130.2 million in 2010. The prevalence is projected to rise to 216.8 million cases by 2020, each with an age-adjusted prevalence of 19.1% (13.9, 25.5), 24.3% (23.3, 31.6) and 25.3% (24.3, 39.7), respectively [54].

In the Heart of Soweto study, among the 1196 persons with the diagnosis of secondary hypertension, 682 or 57% (mean age 60 ± 14 years) had hypertensive HF [16]. In the INTERHEART study, hypertension was reported as a strong contributor to the hazards of CVD in black Africans, with an odd ratio of 7.0 versus 2.3–3.9 in other ethnic groups ($p < 0.0002$) [55].

Hypertension in Africa is associated with body weight, lower intake of potassium and salt sensitivity [56]. The peak age group is 40–49 years. Men are affected more than women. The patterns of presentation of hypertensive HF vary. Some present with acute left ventricular failure and severely elevated blood pressure. A sub-group present with HF and normal blood pressure which tends to rise as the HF is being treated. And yet a third group present with HF and normotension all through. The last group is usually difficult to differentiate from dilated cardiomyopathy in the absence of other signs of long-standing hypertension [57].

The mortality attributable to high blood pressure in most West African Countries ranges between 3 and 7% and cardiovascular mortality is in the range of 20–45% [58]. Women may have added morbidity in Africa if the role of hypertension in pregnancy is factored in. Hypertension is largely asymptomatic until end-organ damage ensues and this is partly responsible for late diagnosis of the disease. Inadequate screening and sub-optimal health facility utilization are also implicated. Therefore, early diagnosis and appropriate therapy would lead to a significant reduction in the prevalence of hypertensive HF in Africa [59].

5.1.2. Rheumatic heart disease (RHD)

It is estimated that 12 million people live with the disease and it results in about 400,000 deaths each year. Two million people will require repeated hospital admission and over a million will need surgery to improve their quality of life. It is common in areas with poor housing condition and an indicator of their plight.

Like hypertension, this was initially thought to be uncommon in Africa [44]. But Cooke in 1901 reported that valvular diseases are common in the continent [3]. This was also supported by reports by other workers [60]. Post-mortem studies have been inconsistent. This may be due to the attitude of Africans towards autopsy.

SSA has a high prevalence of RHD which is in the range of 1–14/1000 children [61–63]. Echocardiography-based population studies report higher prevalence of 7.5–51.6/1000 children [64, 65]. School surveys have given a prevalence of $2.7/10^3$ in Kenya [66], $4.3/10^3$ in Ethiopia [67] and $6.9/10^3$ in South Africa [68] (among black children). Marijon et al. reported a prevalence of $30/10^3$ from an echocardiography-based school survey [69].

RHD accounts for 12–32% of cardiovascular admissions in SSA. Recent reports suggest that that 6.6–34% of CV-related hospital admissions or echocardiographic data in SSA are due to RHD and up to 2.3% of pregnant women have the disease [70–74].

There are peculiar features of rheumatic heart disease in Africa (similar to reports from other tropical environments). These are the young age at presentation, the severity of the lesions, as well as the high mortality associated with it. History of rheumatic fever can be obtained in only less than 50% of patients. Pure mitral incompetence and mixed mitral valve disease were the commonest valvular lesions that were demonstrated [75]. This is consistent with the findings of other workers in Africa [74, 76–78]. A rheumatic carditis has been shown to run a more fulminant course in sub-Saharan Africa (like in other tropical countries) compared to the developed countries [79–82]. In earlier studies, 33% of 124 mitral valvotomies were in patients under the age of 16 years in one report from Kenya.

The disease appears to be commoner in women. Events in women's life such as pregnancy frequently unmask the condition [83]. Morbidity and mortality is said to be high especially in women and young people [83, 84]. Mortality at 6 month is estimated as 17.8% [85]. In one report from Ethiopia, the annual mortality from RHD is as high as 12.5%, and 70% of such deaths were before the age of 26 years [67].

Sliwa et al. [86] reported on the characteristics of 344 adult rheumatic heart disease cases in the Heart of Soweto study. The disease was commoner in black women (68%). The most common valvular lesion (n = 204, 59%) was mitral regurgitation (MR), with 48 (14%) and 43 (13%) cases, respectively, having combination lesions of aortic plus MR and mixed mitral VHD. Impaired systolic function was demonstrated in 28/204 cases (14%) of predominant MR and in 23/126 cases (18%) with predominant aortic regurgitation. The finding from the study makes a case for the first episode of RHD to be made a notifiable condition in high-burden countries in order to ensure control of the disease through register-based secondary prophylaxis programmes.

In many countries in SSA, facilities for accurate diagnosis are unavailable. Treatment options such as valvotomy, valvuloplasty and prosthetic valve replacement are either unavailable or unaffordable to a vast majority of the population. Worse still secondary preventive measures are also either unavailable or unaffordable.

The lack of infrastructure, political, economic and social instability, malnutrition and poverty are all factors implicated in the high prevalence of rheumatic fever in Africa which is, otherwise, largely preventable [80]. This culminates in a great burden of rheumatic valvular heart disease and infective endocarditis.

5.2. The cardiomyopathies

Dilated cardiomyopathy (DCM), endomyocardial fibrosis (EMF) and peripartum cardiomyopathy (PPCM) are common and endemic in SSA. Other forms of cardiomyopathy are less common.

5.2.1. Dilated cardiomyopathy (DCM)

DCM is a major cause of HF in SSA. It has been plagued with diagnostic and therapeutic challenges due to lack of appropriate facilities, definitive diagnosis and interventions in resource-poor African centres. It typically presents with progressive HF and is associated with high mortality. In one study, the 4-year mortality was found to be 34%.

There are marked regional differences in the pathogenesis of dilated cardiomyopathy in Africa. The causative factors that have been implicated in several studies across Africa include infection [87, 88] and myocarditis [89, 90], 'burnt out' untreated hypertension [91], genetic factors, alcohol, nutritional deficiencies, autoimmune mechanisms, iron overload and pregnancy [92].

The current concept is that 30% of the disease has genetic basis. Familial DCM is caused by a mutation in more than 25 chromosome loci. The genes affected are those encoding contractile, cytoskeleton and calcium regulatory proteins.

In 1975, Owor and Rwomushana reported the first case of familial DCM in Africa [93]. They described twin brothers who were affected by the condition in Uganda. Subsequently, other workers have documented familial DCM in other parts of SSA especially from South Africa [94]. However, there are no systematic family studies of the condition in SSA. Some gene association studies have, however, been done especially in South Africa. Some of the findings include:

1. An association with HLADR1 and DRW10 antigens suggesting possible genetically determined immune factors may be responsible for the disease [95, 96].
2. An association with mutation in troponin T-gene (Arg141Trp) [97] and mitochondrial T16185c polymorphism.

On the other hand, there is no evidence of association with cardiac (ACTC1) and skeletal (ACTA1) alpha-actin gene, alpha-2c adrenoceptor (ADRB2c) gene, beta-1 adrenoceptor (ADRB1) gene and tumour necrosis factor-alpha (TNFA) gene.

Some data suggest the immune-modulating agent pentoxifylline may be beneficial in the management of DCM in the region. In one trial, patients on this agent had improvement in effort tolerance, left ventricular function and trend towards lower mortality than those on standard treatment for HF [98].

In a 14-year follow-up of DCM patients in South Africa, a mortality of 10% per year was recorded for both familial and idiopathic DCM. Heart transplantation was an independent predictor of survival, while NYHA III and IV and use of digoxin were associated with poor outcome.

5.2.2. Endomyocardial fibrosis (EMF)

This is a form of restrictive cardiomyopathy in which there is a deposition of fibrous tissue in the mural endocardium resulting in impaired diastolic function as well as valvular dysfunction resulting from entrapment of papillary muscles of the atrioventricular valve. It occurs mainly in the tropical and subtropical areas of Africa. It was first described by William in 1938. It is also called Davies disease because of the seminal work done by Davies on this disorder in Uganda [99–101]. A comprehensive description of the clinical features has been documented by Hutt [102] as well as other workers [103, 104]. Recently, Mocumbi et al. have suggested diagnostic criteria for diagnosis [105].

EMF has been reported in at least 17 SSA countries: Congo, Cameroon, Egypt, Ethiopia, Gabon, Ghana, Kenya, Malawi, Mozambique, Nigeria, Senegal, South Africa, Sudan, Tanzania, Uganda, Zambia and Zimbabwe. It has also been reported in India and South America. It is rare in Northern and Southern Africa. Right-sided EMF appears to be commoner. The peak age incidence is 11–15 year in both sexes. In a population-based study in Mozambique, a prevalence of 8.9% was found.

EMF is a disease of childhood and early adolescence. It has also been reported in older adults and infants. A second peak of incidence has been shown during the reproductive age of women. The preponderance of one gender over the other is inconsistently reported. In a large database from Mozambique, it was reported to be more prevalent in males.

The pathophysiology postulated is as follows: endocardial thickening of the ventricles leads to cardiac constriction or restriction and atrioventricular valvular incompetence resulting in regurgitation. The right ventricular cavity is usually obliterated from below by the advancing fibrosis of layered mural thrombi. In severe and late cases, the papillary muscles are buried in a layer of fibrous tissue leading to functionless tricuspid valve and aneurysmal right atrium. When the left ventricle is involved, dense fibrous tissues are deposited at the apex, spreading around the cavity of the LV or may first appear around the papillary muscles of the posterior cusp of the mitral valve (leading to anchoring of the muscle and valvular regurgitation) [99, 104].

Chronic pericardial effusion commonly complicates right-sided EMF, while pleural effusion is commoner with left or biventricular disease [104]. The clinical features depend on the stage of the disease, the anatomical damage done on the affected valve as well as the resultant effect on heart function. An initial illness with fever, chills, night sweats, facial swelling and urticaria can occur and is reported in 30–50% of cases. This can be fatal within months but little is known about this phase of the disease [104].

In left-sided EMF, the ventricle is not enlarged and there is almost always mitral incompetence and a loud pulmonary component of the second heart sound and progressive pulmonary hypertension. There is usually an early third heat sound. When the right ventricle is involved, the classical picture is that of a young patient with 'egg on stick' or 'orange on stick' appearance (massive ascites and minimal pedal oedema; often with delayed puberty, some exophthalmos and central cyanosis) [104]. The arterial pulse is usually of small volume or feeble. Atrial fibrillation is common. Massive pericardial effusion or a rotated heat (because of massive right atrium) could give an impalpable heart. An abrupt third heart sound is common but murmur may be absent.

The pathogenic process is explained by eosinophil and its constituents. The suggested sequel is as follows [104]:

1. A trigger to eosinophilia (helminthic or other infections and liberation of eosinophilic major basic proteins and cationic proteins which are toxic to the cardiac cells as well as other cells in the body;
2. The damaged endocardium serves as a nidus for thrombus formation;
3. Thrombus formation builds up due to release of platelet-activating factors by the eosinophils;
4. Further mural thrombi are laid down at the original and adjacent sites leading to the formation of fibrotic mass.

Although this explanation appears plausible, it does not offer reason why the disease is rare in some parts of the tropics, the reported ethnic differences [106] and some familial cases of EMF [107].

Despite the fact that the aetiology of this condition has not been resolved by scientist since the first description, the volume of publication on it has dwindled in the last decade. The cause has remained a mystery despite several proposed aetiological factors [108]. Some of the factors that have been implicated in the past include: (1) infections/infestations, for example, cardiotropic viruses, mycoplasma pneumonia, malaria, schistosomiasis, (2) autoimmunity, (3) Hypereosinophilia, (4) genetics and (5) traditional medications.

Trend in the incidence and prevalence of EMF has not been well studied in SSA. Ellis et al. showed that the prevalence has not changed in Uganda [109]. On the other hand, in Nigeria, EMF was shown to have declined from 10% in the 1960/1970s to 0.02% from medical admissions and 0.04% for cardiac-related admissions in the first decade of twenty-first century. This may not be unconnected with improvement in health-care delivery as well as control of communicable diseases in that part of the country [110].

The prognosis of EMF is poor. The survival of patients after diagnosis is about 2 years [104].

5.2.3. *Peripartum cardiomyopathy (PPCM)*

This is defined as heart muscle disease in which left ventricular systolic dysfunction and symptoms of HF occur between the last month of pregnancy and the first 5 months postpartum. In many parts of Africa, the prevalence is about 1/1500 deliveries. However, the northern part of Nigeria appears to be the hot spot for the condition where it affects 1/100 women after delivery. Recent echocardiography-based study from this part of Nigeria confirms similar prevalence [111]. The epidemiology, pathophysiology and clinical features of this condition have been reviewed in detail elsewhere [112–115]. Most patients present within the first 4 months after delivery. Only about 10% present in the last month of pregnancy.

Symptoms and signs are similar to other forms of systolic dysfunction. In addition, they are prone to thromboembolic phenomenon [116].

Aetiological factors implicated include multiparty, advanced maternal age, multiple gestation, preeclampsia, gestational hypertension and black race. Several plausible aetiological mechanisms have been advanced. These include genetic predisposition, myocarditis, cardiotropic viral infections, chimerism, apoptosis and inflammation. Others include abnormal haemodynamic response, immune complexes, cardiac nitric oxide synthase, immune dendritic cells, cardiac dystrophin, etc. [113, 117].

A novel molecular mechanism of PPCM has been documented. Such mechanisms include elevated pro-inflammatory markers such as sFas/Apo 1, interferon-gamma, interleukin-6 and C-reactive protein. These points to the pro-inflammatory mechanism in the initiation, progression and prognosis of the disease. A pathophysiological circuit that involves unbalanced oxidative stress which leads to enhanced cleavage of prolactin into pro-apoptotic and angiogenic 16-kDa sub-fragments has been described. This process results in endothelial damage and LV dysfunction. Presence of endothelial damage in PPCM is further supported by the presence of endothelial microparticles suggesting apoptosis with impaired microcirculation. Furthermore, the angiogenic imbalance in this condition may also be contributed by soluble fms-like tyrosine kinase [118].

About 23–54% of PPCM patients have normalization of LV function at 6 months. Poor outcome is associated with increased LV systolic dimension, lower body mass index and low serum cholesterol at the time of presentation. On the other hand, older age and smaller LV end-systolic diameter is associated with higher chances of recovery of LV function [118].

The mortality associated with PPCM is 15% at 6 months, 28% at 2 years and 42% in over 25 years of follow-up. Predictors of mortality include NYHA functional class at presentation, cardiothoracic ratio, electrocardiographic QRS duration and higher diastolic pressure [119, 120]. A proof-of-concept pilot study has provided some evidence of the benefit of bromocriptine in PPCM patients [121].

5.2.4. Other cardiomyopathies

5.2.4.1. Hypertrophic cardiomyopathy

Earlier reports of this condition were mainly anecdotal and it was generally thought to be uncommon in Africa. The earliest report appears to be that of Lewis et al. in 1973 [122]. Thereafter, other reports followed [123–127]. In 1240 consecutive echocardiography in Ethiopia, the prevalence of HCM was 4.3% (54 subjects) and accounted for 34.4% of cardiomyopathies [128]. In a similar study in Tanzania, it accounted for 0.2% of 6680 echocardiograms [129]. HCM is the third commonest cardiomyopathy in Ghana [13].

The genetic studies done on this condition have emanated only from South Africa where facilities are available [130–139]. The disease-causing genetic mutation or loci has been documented. These include beta-myosin heavy chain (MYH7) gene, myosin binding protein c (MYBPC3) gene and troponin T (TNNT2) gene. Carriers of T (TNNT2) R92W mutation develop cardiac hypertrophy after the age of 35 years. They also have abnormal response to exercise which may explain the high mortality associated with this mutation [140].

The physiological effects of genetic mutations that cause HCM have also been studied in the continent. TNNT R92W mutation is associated with a relative increase in LV systolic functional parameters. Reduced diastolic function has been demonstrated in MYH7 A797T mutation, while MYH7 R403W mutation is associated with reduction in both systolic and diastolic functions [141, 142].

Furthermore, angiotensin II type 2 receptor (AGTR2) gene and angiotensin converting enzyme 2 (ACE2) gene have been identified as genetic risk factors (i.e. genetic polymorphism with evidence of association with HCM) [130, 143].

5.2.4.2. Arrhythmogenic right ventricular cardiomyopathy (ARVC)

The first report of ARVC from the region was in the year 2000 [144]. Kindred that are linked to ARVC type 6 locus have been documented [145]. The first multicentre registry of ARVC was reported from South Africa [146]. Data from the registry show that the disease occurs in all racial and ethnic groups in the country. Symptoms start from the third decade of life and the most common symptoms are palpitation, dizziness, syncope and chest pain. Symptoms are more pronounced in males. The reported male to female ratio is 2:1. About 28% were professional endurance athletes at some point in their lives. About 30% of the participants have family members who are also affected and 25% had plakophilin-2 gene defect [146, 147].

Interestingly, the rare 'allele-dose-defect' was demonstrated in one of the subjects, while haplotype analysis also demonstrated the uncommon 'founder effect' in many of the subjects [146, 147].

The annual mortality is 2.8% and 5-year cumulative mortality is 10% [146, 147].

5.2.4.3. Isolated left ventricular non-compaction (ILVNC)

Ker et al. [148] reported the first case of ILVNC in SSA in 2006. Since then, there have been reports from Djibouti [149], South Africa [150, 151] Sudan [152] and Nigeria [153]. The disorder is a common cause of HF, disorders of cardiac rhythm and cardioembolism and is as a result of failure of the myocardium to compact in utero.

In a series comprising of 54-ILVNC patients, Peters et al. [150] in Johannesburg showed that the prevalence is 6.9% and the mean age of presentation is 45.4 ± 13.1 years. It occurs commonly in males (55.6%) and majority (63.0%) present in NYHA class II. HF with systolic dysfunction is the common mode of presentation (98.1%). The identified sites of non-compaction include apical (100%), mid-inferior (74.1%) and mid-lateral walls (64.8%). The disorder has also been documented to be associated with pulmonary hypertension (83.3%), right ventricular (RV) dilation (74.1%) and impaired RV function (59.3%).

5.2.4.4. HIV-associated cardiomyopathy

This is another cause of HF in Africa. Globally, the prevalence was 2–40% in the pre-highly active anti-retroviral treatment (Pre-HAART) era [154, 155]. However, with the introduction of HAART, the prevalence has fallen in many parts of the world. But in some parts of SSA, due to poverty, ignorance, weak health system, malnutrition and low utility of HAART, the high of HIV-associated cardiomyopathy is prevalent. The effectiveness of HAART is also supported by data from Uganda that showed low prevalence of this condition in children on this treatment [156].

The true prevalence of HIV-associated cardiomyopathy is unknown in the sub-region. Prevalence from reported literature ranges from 5% in Nigeria to 57% in Burkina Faso [157–159]. It is the commonest cardiac diagnosis in HIV-infected people in the Heart of Soweto study and more common in those with high viral load and lower CD4 count [160].

6. Pericardial diseases

Pericarditis and pericardial effusion are common in SSA and are frequently a cause of HF in the region. In some areas, over 15% of cardiovascular admission may be due to primary pericardial diseases. Tuberculosis is the leading cause of pericardial disease in Africa and this is often complicated by constrictive pericarditis. The burden of pericardial disease in SSA has escalated due to the impact of HIV/AIDS.

Next to tuberculosis is purulent pericarditis secondary to streptococcal or staphylococcal infection. Viruses may be responsible for most cases of benign pericarditis without demonstrable aetiology. Other causes include parasitic infections such as trypanosomiasis and malaria.

7. Congenital heart disease

Few publications have looked at cardiovascular disease in young Africans despite the fact that two-thirds of the population of SSA are made up of children and young adults. Congenital heart diseases constitute about 0.3% of heart diseases seen in northern Nigeria [161] to 12% in the series documented by Bertrand in Ivory Coast [162]. The high value in the later may be because the centre at a time served a large referral centre for cardiac surgery in West Africa.

A prevalence of 13.1% was documented in Cameroon (mean age: 10 ± 9 years, range: 2 months–41 years) [163]. About 35% of children with HF in Uganda have congenital heart disease [109].

To the best of our knowledge, the only population-based data on congenital heart disease is from Mozambique where the prevalence was reported as 2.3/1000 children [164].

The pattern of cardiac lesions appears not to be different from reports from other parts of the world in terms of the most frequent lesions. In the decreasing order of frequency, ventricular septal defect, atrial septal defect, Fallot's tetralogy and patent ductus arteriosus are the common congenital heart diseases that may lead to cardiac failure in Africa [164–179]. Recognition of cyanosis in the dark skin may pose a challenge coupled with the fact that anaemia is common in SSA population.

Lack of trained man power, scarcity of diagnostic tools as well as poverty mitigates the care of patients with congenital heart disease in the region.

http://dx.doi.org/10.5772/intechopen.82416

8. Coronary artery disease

It is generally believed that coronary artery disease is uncommon in SSA. However, recent reports emanating from the region suggest that the disease is emerging, and when it occurs, the clinical as well as the pathological features are similar to that seen in Caucasians [180]. In early reports, Edington [181] in 1954 noted only 3 cases in about 3500 consecutive autopsies in present-day Ghana. Sharper and Williams [5] documented nine cases seen in Uganda over a 3-year period (1955–1957). Falase et al. [182] reported 26 cases over a period spanning 1961–1970 and calculated a prevalence rate of 1:20,500 for Ibadan, Nigeria. In another study by the same author, the prevalence has increased to 1:10,000. Okuwobi [183] saw seven cases over a period of 3 years. Bertrand [184] reported 75 cases over a 6-year period and this accounted for 0.83% of total cardiac-related admission.

Recent reports still report low prevalence of this condition but the trend is that it is on the increase. In a study of HF in elderly subjects (60 years and above), Ikama and his colleagues reported a prevalence of 25.6% in this age group [185].

Studies done in South Africa between 1992 and 2008 show remarkable increase in the prevalence of the disease. In 1994, the prevalence was 0.2% [186] but the recent report from the Heart of Soweto study shows a prevalence of about 10%. This is remarkable evidence of gradual shift in disease pattern (epidemiologic transition) in this population. The prevalence reported in earlier studies ranged from 0.4 to 1.0% [187–189].

9. Pulmonary heart disease (cor pulmonale) and pulmonary hypertension

This is also emerging as a common cause of heart disease in SSA. In the Heart of Soweto study, right HF or cor pulmonale was documented in 27% of individuals admitted for HF. The prevalence in other regions is as follows: 0.8–9.5% in West Africa and 0.3–7.7% in Eastern Africa.

At least six reports have looked at the aetiology of pulmonary heart disease in SSA [190–195]. The common aetiological factors described include left heart disease, chronic obstructive pulmonary disease, bronchiectasis, tuberculosis, bronchial asthma, pulmonary fibrosis of unknown origin, pulmonary embolism (acute cor pulmonale), HIV/AIDs and thromboembolic obliterative pulmonary hypertension.

Tuberculosis and chronic obstructive pulmonary disease is the major culprit. The situation is worsened by the emergence of HIV/AIDS. Globally, there has been an increase in the incidence of tuberculosis by 2.2 million from 1997 to 2005 and 95% of this is occurring in developing countries. In a recent autopsy report from South Africa, it was reported that 31% of cases had pulmonary hypertension as cause or part of their cardiac lesion.

HIV-associated pulmonary hypertension is being increasingly reported in SSA [196]. Hakim et al. [197] and Niakara et al. [158] recently reported a prevalence of 5%. Other causes of pulmonary hypertension in SSA include sickle cell anaemia [198], connective tissue disease, congenital heart disease [199], valvular heart disease [74], schistosomiasis [200, 201], laryngeal papillomatosis [202], sarcoma [203], herbal remedies [204], hypertensive disorders of pregnancy [205], vaso-occlusive disorders [206] and primary pulmonary hypertension [207].

10. Gender differences

In the THESUS HF registry, men were significantly older and presented in poorer NYHA functional class. Men are also more likely to be current or previous smokers and have higher blood pressure. Renal dysfunction, poorer left ventricular ejection fraction and higher transmitral E/A ratio are also more frequent in men. Atrial fibrillation, anaemia and valvular heart disease are significantly more common in women [216].

11. Regional differences

Hypertensive HF as aetiological risk factor for HF is less reported in countries in the horn of Africa, for example, Ethiopia, Eritrea and Djibouti contrary to reports from west and central Africa [18]. Ischaemic heart disease is now the commonest cause of HF in Sudan (an example of country undergoing rapid epidemiologic transition; see **Figure 3**) This explains the difference in the picture presented by the THESUS HF survey [27] and the African data in the INTER-CHF study [26, 40]. Data from Nigeria and Sudan predominated in the two studies, respectively. Cardiomyopathy appears to be commoner in southern and eastern (except Tanzania) parts of the continent. HIV-associated cardiomyopathy has been commonly reported from the southern region of the continent (**Figure 4A–D**).

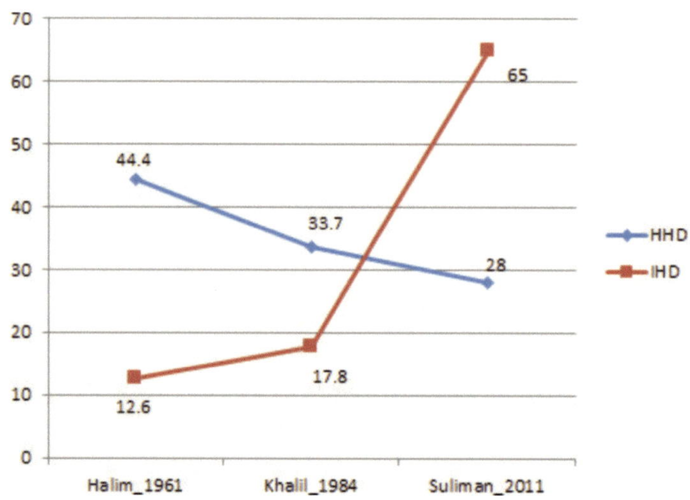

Figure 3. Sudan epidemiologic transition.

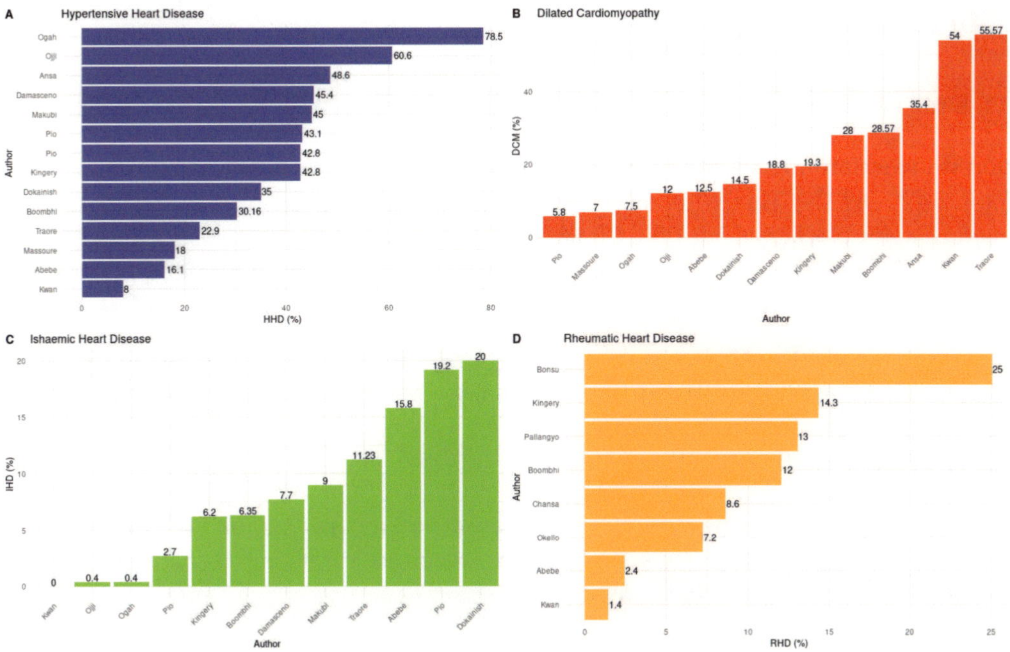

Figure 4. Spectrum of aetiology of HF in various studies in SSA.

12. Laboratory findings

12.1. 12-Lead ECG

ECG abnormalities are common in patients with HF in SSA [217, 218]. The common major ECG abnormalities are left ventricular hypertrophy, inverted T-wave, atrial fibrillation, Q waves compatible with myocardial infarction, premature ventricular and supraventricular beats and bundle branch blocks. Common minor abnormalities are axis deviation, ST-T changes, ST elevation, isolated pathological Q-wave and right ventricular hypertrophy [218].

In the THESUS HF study, a higher ventricular was associated with higher 180-day readmission or mortality. QRS duration and corrected QT interval were not associated with either composite of death or readmission through 60 days or death through 180 days [218].

12.2. Echocardiography

About 70% of HF patients in SSA have LV ejection fraction lower than 40% [17–19, 27]. This is associated with male gender, presence of pedal oedema, higher heart rate, lower blood pressure and renal dysfunction. Left atrial size among other clinical variables predicts rehospitalisation or death within 60 days. Left ventricular posterior wall added to clinical variables predicts 180-day mortality rates [219]. The recently described mid-range ejection fraction has not been fully described in Africa. In a recent retrospective report from Ghana, the distribution of HFrEF, HFmrEF and HFpEF are 23.2, 17.8 and 59%, respectively [220].

13. In-hospital care

13.1. Drug treatment

Loop diuretics are the commonest medication used for the treatment of HF in SSA (81.6, 95% CI: 72.7–89.1%) This is followed by angiotensin-converting enzyme inhibitors/angiotensin receptor blockers (75%, 95% CI: 64.4–85.1%), aldosterone antagonists (51.5%, 95% CI: 32.4–70%), beta-blockers (31.4%, 95% CI: 22.6–40.9%) and digoxin (31.5%, 95% CI: 19.4–45%) [221, 222].

The use of nitrates is low (7.9%). Parenteral inotropes (dopamine and dobutamine) are uncommonly used (5.0 and 5.1%, respectively). Mechanical ventilation is rarely used (0.6%) [27].

13.2. Procedural investigations

Unlike in developed countries, the use of procedural investigations is not well documented in SSA. This is most likely due to limited access to these procedures, high cost as well as limited reports from various centres in the region.

14. Co-morbidities

14.1. Renal dysfunction

About 7.7–48% of HF patients in SSA have renal dysfunction. Worsening renal function occurs in about 10% of cases. This is commoner in West Africa. It is also associated with overweight/obesity and presence of basal crackles at admission. Presence of renal dysfunction is also independently associated with higher readmission rate over 60 days and all-cause mortality over 180 days [36].

14.2. Atrial fibrillation

In the THESUS HF survey, atrial fibrillation (AF) was documented in about 20%. Individuals with AF are older than the general HF population; they are more likely to be females and they have significantly higher heart rate but lower blood pressure. Presence of AF is not associated with poorer outcome; however, valvular AF is associated with all-cause readmission and mortality [223]. AF is associated with poorer outcome in Tanzania [19].

14.3. Anaemia

Rates of anaemia range from 8% in Abuja Nigeria to 64.3% in Uganda. Higher rates have been recorded in other East African countries and northern Nigeria [224, 225]. Iron deficiency anaemia occurs in about 57% of HF patients in Tanzania. This has been shown to be associated with poor prognosis. **Table 2** shows the prevalence of anaemia in some SSA countries.

Authors	Country	Year	Number	% Anaemia	Definition
Makubi [19]	Tanzania	2014	427	57	<10 g/dl
Ogah [18]	Nigeria (South)	2014	452	8.8	<10 g/dl
Damasceno [27]	Multi-country	2012	1006	15.2	<10 g/dl
Stewart [17]	South Africa	2008	699	10.0	Male, <11 g/dl, female <10 g/dl
Karaye [226]	Nigeria (North)	2008	100	45%	NA
Kuule [227]	Uganda	2009	157	64.3	Male, ≤12.9 g/dl, female, ≤11.9 g/dl
Inglis [233]	South Africa	2007	163	13.5	WHO
Dzudie [234]	Cameroon	2008	140	15.7	NA

NA = not available.

Table 2. Prevalence of anaemia in some HF studies in SSA.

14.4. Psychological dysfunction and depression

Psychological distress is common in SSA patients with HF. More than one-third (39%) have both depression and anxiety while about 16 and 13% have depression and anxiety respectively. Furthermore, two-thirds of in-patients and one-third of out-patients have depression [226, 227]. Psychological distress and depression is more common in young HF patients because of challenges of coping and adjusting with the condition [228].

14.5. Heart failure knowledge and compliance to treatment

HF patients in Africa have poor knowledge of their illness, the medications and side effects. The compliance to medications is also poor especially with diuretics because of the side effects. Ability to recall medications is also poor [229, 230].

15. Outcomes

15.1. Length of hospital stay

The median length of hospital stay ranges from 7 days in the THESUS HF survey, 11 days in Abeokuta, Nigeria and 13 days in a rural health facility in the Cameroun.

15.2. Readmission rate

Readmission after an initial or index case of HF is common, and CV reasons (worsening HF) are responsible in most of the cases. The rate of readmission or death at 60 days is about 15.4%.

15.3. Mortality

15.3.1. In-hospital mortality

The reported in-hospital mortality is in the range of 3.8–25.2% (see **Figure 5**) [18, 20, 24, 27, 29, 30, 233].

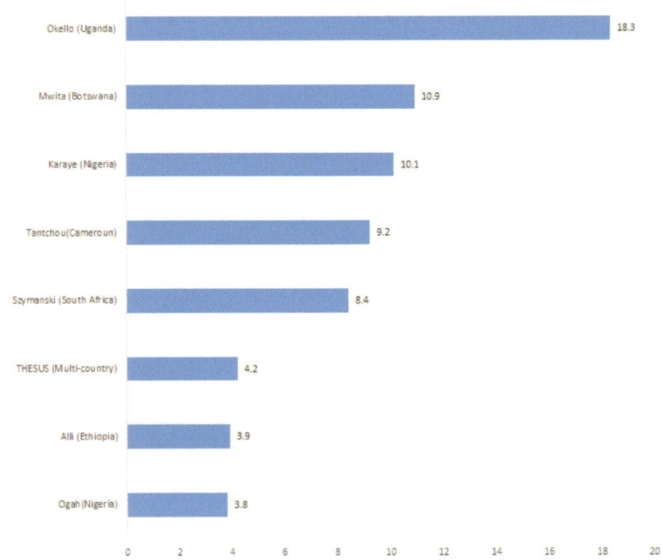

Figure 5. Intra-hospital mortality from various HF studies in SSA.

15.3.2. Short- and medium-term mortality

Thirty-day mortality rate ranges from 14.7 to 35% [221, 234]. The reported 60- and 180-days readmission or mortality is 15–57.8 and 21.9–57.9%, respectively. Common predictors of readmission or mortality include presence of malignancy, severe lung disease, admission for blood pressure, heart rate, signs of congestion, renal function and ejection fraction. Others include anaemia, history of smoking and HIV co-infection [221, 234].

15.3.3. Long-term mortality

A 3-year mortality rate of 67.1% was reported in patients with advanced heart failure from one centre in Nigeria [212]. In a recent retrospective report from Ghana, the 1-, 2- and 5-year survival rates were reported as 90.3, 64.7 and 38.4%, respectively. Those with HFpEF are older, are more often women and often have non-ischaemic etiology for the HF. They also have higher rates of CKD and atrial fibrillation but lower rates of DCM. On the other hand, those with HFrEF are more symptomatic and are more likely to receive disease-modifying medications [220]. Among individuals with HFpEF, anaemia, DCM, diabetes mellitus, presence of cerebrovascular event, use of statin and aldosterone antagonist independently predicted mortality. On the other hand, severe HF symptoms, history of smoking and use of beta-blockers were independent predictors of death in HFmrEF patients. Age is a predictor of mortality in all the three HF groups. HFpEF has a better long-term prognosis [220].

15.4. Quality of life (QoL) and spiritual well-being

Poor quality of life has been demonstrated in over 25% of HF patients in Nigeria. Age and educational attainment are major determinants of QoL [235]. In Kenya, spiritual distress is common and more often in younger patients [236].

http://dx.doi.org/10.5772/intechopen.82416

15.5. Economic cost

In developing countries, about 15.1 billion US dollars was spent on the care of HF in the year 2012 [237]. The cost of HF in Nigeria in the year 2009 was estimated at 508,595 USD, translating to 2128 USD per patient per year. In-patient and out-patient care cost constituted 46 and 54% of total care cost, respectively. The relatively higher cost of out-patient care cost was attributed to the cost of transportation for monthly follow-up visits. Payment for the care of HF is out-of-pocket in most parts of SSA.

16. Comparison with other parts of the world

Compared to other regions of the world, HF patients in SSA are younger. The mean age in the THESUS HF survey [27] was 52 years compared to 69.9 years in the EURO HF survey, 72.4 years in the ADHERE study (in USA, 71 years in Japan and 60 years in Indonesia; **Table 3**) [27].

They are more likely to have rheumatic heart disease as the aetiology, while ischemic heart disease is less likely. They are also relatively less likely to have diabetes mellitus, atrial fibrillation and chronic obstructive airway disease as co-morbidity. The prevalence of chronic kidney disease and anaemia is lower in SSA HF patients. The mean left ventricular EF and median length of hospital stay appear to be similar to other parts of the world [27]. In the INTER-CHF study, the age-adjusted mortality is worse in SSA compared to other low- and middle-income regions [27].

17. Gaps and future directions

There is generally no population-based incidence or prevalence data on HF in SSA. The community or population-based data on the burden of systolic or diastolic dysfunction using echocardiography is unknown. In addition, apart from high blood pressure, the community burden of other aetiological risk factors for HF such as EMF, rheumatic heart disease and right HF is largely scanty.

The molecular pathobiology of HF in SSA is largely unexplored. The secular trend in HF in SSA is also unknown. This has been well studied in high-income countries of Europe and North America. There is also need for research into best strategies for treatment and prevention of common causes of HF in the region. More cohort studies and longer follow-up of HF patients are needed in SSA to fully describe the natural history of HF. An in-depth cost analysis or economic analysis as well as data on quality of care is also scanty and needs exploring. Clinical trials on HF are generally lacking.

Finally, in-depth scientific approaches to better understand the epidemiology, pathobiology, socio-cultural factors, treatment patterns as well as outcome of HF and diseases leading to HF should be the focus of future research. As suggested by Fonn, 'research conceptualized, conducted, analysed and published by Africans is crucial for Africa to meet the health needs of her people' [238].

Study	No	% Women	Mean age	Smoking	Hypertension	Diabetes	Anaemia	CKD	NYHA (III & IV)	Mean EF	HHF	DCM	VHDX	RHF	IHD	LOS	M
THESUS_ HF^{S} [27]	1006	50.7	52	9.8	55.5	11.1	15.2	7.7	34.6	39.5	45.4	18.8	14.3	NR	7.7	7	4.2
EuroHeart failure [243]	3580	38.7	69.9	NR	62.5	32.8	14.7	16.8	NR	38	11.4	19.3		3.2	53.6	9	6.7
ADHERE, USA	105,388	52	72.4	NR	73	44	NR	30	76	34.4						4.3	4
OPTIMIZE, USA	48,612	52	73	NR	NR	NR	NR	NR	NR	39							3.8
ADHERE, Indonesia	1687	64.5	60	74	54.8	31.2	NR	NR	NR	37.9	54.8	NR	NR	NR	23.3	7.1	6.7
JCARE-CARD, Japan	2675	40.3	71	37.7	52.9	29.9	20.8	11.7	87.5	42.2	24.6	21.9	15.7	NR	32	NR	NR

EF = ejection fraction, NYHA = New York Heart Association, CKD = chronic kidney disease, HHF = hypertensive heart failure, DCM = dilated cardiomyopathy, VHDX = valvular heart disease, RHF = right heart failure, IHD = ischaemic heart disease, LOS = length of stay in hospital, M = intra-hospital mortality.

Table 3. Comparison of present study with other HF studies in SSA and other parts of the world.

18. Conclusions

African HF patients are the youngest compared to most regions of the world. They are most likely to be illiterate and often lack medication or health insurance. They are most likely to be in the worst NYHA functional class and less likely to be on any beta-blocker.

Hypertensive heart disease is the commonest aetiological risk factor. Other risk factors include dilated cardiomyopathy, rheumatic heart disease and ischaemic heart disease. HF-related mortality is also high in SSA.

Author details

Okechukwu S. Ogah[1]*, Adewole Adebiyi[1] and Karen Sliwa[2,3,4]

*Address all correspondence to: osogah56156@gmail.com

1 Division of Cardiology, Department of Medicine, University College Hospital/University of Ibadan, Ibadan, Nigeria

2 Hatter Institute for Cardiovascular Research in Africa, Department of Medicine and Cardiology, Faculty of Health Sciences, University of Cape Town, Cape Town, South Africa

3 Soweto Cardiovascular Research Unit, Faculty of Health Sciences, University of the Witwatersrand, Johannesbure, South Africa

4 Mary MacKillop Institute for Health Research, Australian Catholic University, Australia

References

[1] United Nations. World Population Prospects: The 2006 Revision Population Database. 2006. Available from: www.un.org/esa/population/publications/wpp2006/English.pdf

[2] Sub-Saharan Africa. Wikipedia: The Free Encyclopedia. 2009. Available from: http://en.wikipedia.org/wiki/Sub-Saharan_Africa

[3] Cooke A. Notes on the disease met with in Uganda, Central Africa. Journal of Tropical Medicine. 1901;**4**:175-178

[4] Vaughan JP. A brief review of cardiovascular disease in Africa. Transactions of the Royal Society of Tropical Medicine and Hygiene. 1977;**71**(3):226-231

[5] Shaper AG, Williams AW. Cardiovascular disorders at an African hospital in Uganda. Transactions of the Royal Society of Tropical Medicine and Hygiene. 1960;**54**:12-32

[6] Shaper AG, Shaper L. Analysis of medical admissions to Mulago Hospital, 1957. East African Medical Journal. 1958;**35**(12):647-678

[7] Lauckner JR, Rankin AM, Adi FC. Analysis of medical admissions to the University College Hospital Ibadan. West African Journal of Medicine. 1961;**10**:3-32

[8] Turner PP. The pattern of disease as seen by medical admissions to the Coast Province General Hospital in 1960. East African Medical Journal. 1962;**39**:121-135

[9] Nhonoli AM. Heart disease in Dar es Salaam. East African Medical Journal. 1968; **45**(3):118-121

[10] Brown KG, Willis WH. Cardiac disease in Malawi. South African Medical Journal. 1975;**49**(23):926-930

[11] Edginton ME, Hodkinson J, Seftel HC. Disease patterns in a South African rural Bantu population, including a commentary on comparisons with the pattern in urbanized Johannesburg Bantu. South African Medical Journal. 1972;**46**(28):968-976

[12] Oyoo GO, Ogola EN. Clinical and socio demographic aspects of congestive heart failure patients at Kenyatta National Hospital, Nairobi. East African Medical Journal. 1999; **76**(1):23-27

[13] Amoah AG, Kallen C. Aetiology of heart failure as seen from a National Cardiac Referral Centre in Africa. Cardiology. 2000;**93**(1-2):11-18

[14] Kingue S et al. A new look at adult chronic heart failure in Africa in the age of the Doppler echocardiography: Experience of the medicine department at Yaounde General Hospital. Annales de Cardiologie et d'Angéiologie (Paris). 2005;**54**(5):276-283

[15] Ojji DB et al. Pattern of heart failure in Abuja, Nigeria: An echocardiographic study. Cardiovascular Journal of Africa. 2009;**20**(6):349-352

[16] Sliwa K et al. Spectrum of heart disease and risk factors in a black urban population in South Africa (the Heart of Soweto Study): A cohort study. Lancet. 2008;**371**(9616): 915-922

[17] Stewart S et al. Predominance of heart failure in the Heart of Soweto Study cohort: Emerging challenges for urban African communities. Circulation. 2008;**118**(23):2360-2367

[18] Ogah OS et al. Contemporary profile of acute heart failure in Southern Nigeria: Data from the Abeokuta Heart Failure Clinical Registry. JACC: Heart Failure. 2014;**2**(3):250-259

[19] Makubi A et al. Contemporary aetiology, clinical characteristics and prognosis of adults with heart failure observed in a tertiary hospital in Tanzania: The prospective Tanzania Heart Failure (TaHeF) study. Heart. 2014;**100**(16):1235-1241

[20] Okello S et al. Characteristics of acute heart failure hospitalizations in a general medical ward in Southwestern Uganda. International Journal of Cardiology. 2014;**176**(3): 1233-1234

[21] Boombhi J et al. Clinical pattern and outcome of acute heart failure at the Yaounde Central Hospital. Open Access Library Journal. 2017;**4**(03):1

[22] Osuji CU et al. Pattern of cardiovascular admissions at Nnamdi Azikiwe University Teaching Hospital Nnewi, South East Nigeria. The Pan African Medical Journal. 2014;**17**:116-121

[23] Massoure PL et al. Heart failure patterns in Djibouti: epidemiologic transition. Medecine et Sante Tropicales. 2013;**23**(2):211-216

[24] Mwita JC et al. Presentation and mortality of patients hospitalised with acute heart failure in Botswana. Cardiovascular Journal of Africa. 2017;**28**(2):112

[25] Abebe TB et al. Patients with HFpEF and HFrEF have different clinical characteristics but similar prognosis: A retrospective cohort study. BMC Cardiovascular Disorders. 2016;**16**(1):232

[26] Dokainish H et al. Heart failure in Africa, Asia, the Middle East and South America: The INTER-CHF study. International Journal of Cardiology. 2016;**204**:133-141

[27] Damasceno A et al. The causes, treatment, and outcome of acute heart failure in 1006 Africans from 9 countries. Archives of Internal Medicine. 2012;**172**(18):1386-1394

[28] Pio M et al. Epidemiology and etiology of heart failure in Lome. The Pan African Medical Journal. 2014;**18**:183

[29] Kingery JR et al. Heart failure, post-hospital mortality and renal function in Tanzania: A prospective cohort study. International Journal of Cardiology. 2017;**243**:311-317

[30] Ali K, Workicho A, Gudina EK. Hyponatremia in patients hospitalized with heart failure: A condition often overlooked in low-income settings. International Journal of General Medicine. 2016;**9**:267-273

[31] Adeoti AO et al. Pattern and outcome of medical admissions in Ekiti state university teaching hospital, Ado-Ekiti-a 5 year review. American Journal of Medicine and Medical Sciences. 2015;**5**(2):92-98

[32] Pio M et al. Young heart failure: Epidemiological, clinical and etiological aspects in the teaching hospital Sylvanus Olympio of Lome. Annales de Cardiologie et d'Angéiologie (Paris). 2014;**63**(4):240-244

[33] Chansa P et al. Factors associated with mortality in adults admitted with heart failure at the University Teaching Hospital in Lusaka, Zambia. Medical Journal of Zambia. 2014;**41**(1):4-12

[34] Ogah OS et al. Spectrum of heart diseases in a new cardiac service in Nigeria: An echocardiographic study of 1441 subjects in Abeokuta. BMC Research Notes. 2008;**1**(1):98

[35] Traore F et al. Heart failure with preserved ejection fraction: A report about 64 cases followed at the Heart Institute of Abidjan. World Journal of Cardiovascular Diseases. 2017;**7**(09):285

[36] Sani MU et al. Renal dysfunction in African patients with acute heart failure. European Journal of Heart Failure. 2014;**16**(7):718-728

[37] Sliwa K et al. Readmission and death after an acute heart failure event: Predictors and outcomes in sub-Saharan Africa: Results from the THESUS-HF registry. European Heart Journal. 2013;**34**(40):3151-3159

[38] Pallangyo P et al. Cardiorenal anemia syndrome and survival among heart failure patients in Tanzania: A prospective cohort study. BMC Cardiovascular Disorders. 2017; **17**(1):59

[39] Kwan GF et al. A simplified echocardiographic strategy for heart failure diagnosis and management within an integrated noncommunicable disease clinic at district hospital level for sub-Saharan Africa. JACC: Heart Failure. 2013;**1**(3):230-236

[40] Dokainish H et al. Heart failure in low- and middle-income countries: Background, rationale, and design of the INTERnational Congestive Heart Failure study (INTER-CHF). American Heart Journal. 2015;**170**(4):627-634 e1

[41] Kimani K et al. What is known about heart failure in sub-Saharan Africa: A scoping review of the English literature. BMJ Supportive & Palliative Care. 2017;**7**:122-127

[42] Carlson S et al. Capacity for diagnosis and treatment of heart failure in sub-Saharan Africa. Heart. 2017;**103**(23):1874-1879

[43] Laabes EP, Thacher TD, Okeahialam BN. Risk factors for heart failure in adult Nigerians. Acta Cardiologica. 2008;**63**(4):437-443

[44] Donnison C. Blood pressure in the African natives: Its bearing upon aetiology of hyperplasia and arteriosclerosis. Lancet. 1929;**1**:6-7

[45] Jex-Blake AJ. High blood pressure. East African Medical Journal. 1934;**10**:286-300

[46] Vint FW. Postmortem findings in natives of Kenya. East African Medical Journal. 1937; **13**:332-340

[47] Williams AW. The blood pressure of the Africans. East African Medical Journal. 1941; **18**:109-117

[48] Davies JN. Pathology of Central African natives; Mulago Hospital post mortem studies. East African Medical Journal. 1948;**25**(12):454-467

[49] Becker B. Cardiovascular disease in the Bantu and coloured races of South Africa. The South African Journal of Medical Sciences. 1946;**11**:1-107

[50] Akinkugbe OO, Nicholson GD, Cruickshank JK. Heart disease in blacks of Africa and the Caribbean. Cardiovascular Clinics. 1991;**21**(3):377-391

[51] Opie LH. Heart disease in Africa. Lancet. 2006;**368**(9534):449-450

[52] Akosa AB, Armah H. Cardiomegaly in Ghana: An autopsy study. Ghana Medical Journal. 2005;**39**(4):122-127

[53] Cooper RS, Amoah AG, Mensah GA. High blood pressure: The foundation for epidemic cardiovascular disease in African populations. Ethnicity & Disease. 2003;**13**(Suppl 2): S48-S52

[54] Adeloye D. An estimate of the incidence and prevalence of stroke in Africa: A systematic review and meta-analysis. PLoS One. 2014;**9**(6):e100724

[55] Steyn K et al. Risk factors associated with myocardial infarction in Africa: The INTERHEART Africa study. Circulation. 2005;**112**(23):3554-3561

[56] Seedat YK. Perspectives of hypertension in black patients: Black vs. white differences. Journal of Cardiovascular Pharmacology. 1990;**16**(Suppl 7):S67-S70

[57] Araoye MA, Olowoyeye O. The clinical spectrum of hypertensive heart failure: A point-score system for solving an old problem. East African Medical Journal. 1984;**61**(4): 306-315

[58] Muna WF. Cardiovascular disorders in Africa. World Health Statistics Quarterly. 1993; **46**(2):125-133

[59] Dzudie A et al. Roadmap to achieve 25% hypertension control in Africa by 2025. Global Heart. 2018;**13**(1):45-59

[60] Heinmann HL. Cardiac disease among African Non-Europeans. British Medical Journal. 1929;**i**:344

[61] Marijon E et al. Prevalence of rheumatic heart disease detected by echocardiographic screening. The New England Journal of Medicine. 2007;**357**(5):470-476

[62] Carapetis JR, McDonald M, Wilson NJ. Acute rheumatic fever. Lancet. 2005;**366**(9480): 155-168

[63] Kimbally-Kaky G et al. Rheumatic heart disease in schoolchildren in Brazzaville. Medecine Tropicale (Mars). 2008;**68**(6):603-605

[64] Beaton A et al. Echocardiography screening for rheumatic heart disease in Ugandan schoolchildren. Circulation. 2012;**125**(25):3127-3132

[65] Kane A et al. Echocardiographic screening for rheumatic heart disease: Age matters. International Journal of Cardiology. 2013;**168**(2):888-891

[66] Anabwani GM, Bonhoeffer P. Prevalence of heart disease in school children in rural Kenya using colour-flow echocardiography. East African Medical Journal. 1996;**73**(4):215-217

[67] Oli K, Asmera J. Rheumatic heart disease in Ethiopia: Could it be more malignant. Ethiopian Medical Journal. 2004;**42**(1):1-8

[68] McLaren MJ et al. Epidemiology of rheumatic heart disease in black shcool children of Soweto, Johannesburg. British Medical Journal. 1975;**3**(5981):474-478

[69] Marijon E et al. Echocardiographic screening for rheumatic heart disease. Bulletin of the World Health Organization. 2008;**86**(2):84

[70] Tantchou Tchoumi JC et al. Occurrence, aetiology and challenges in the management of congestive heart failure in sub-Saharan Africa: Experience of the cardiac Centre in Shisong, Cameroon. The Pan African Medical Journal. 2011;**8**:11

[71] Tantchou Tchoumi JC, Butera G. Rheumatic valvulopathies occurence, pattern and follow-up in rural area: The experience of the Shisong Hospital, Cameroon. Bulletin de la Société de Pathologie Exotique. 2009;**102**(3):155-158

[72] Soliman EZ, Juma H. Cardiac disease patterns in northern Malawi: Epidemiologic transition perspective. Journal of Epidemiology. 2008;**18**(5):204-208

[73] Ike SO. Echocardiographic analysis of valvular heart diseases over one decade in Nigeria. Transactions of the Royal Society of Tropical Medicine and Hygiene. 2008; **102**(12):1214-1218

[74] Sani MU, Karaye KM, Borodo MM. Prevalence and pattern of rheumatic heart disease in the Nigerian savannah: An echocardiographic study. Cardiovascular Journal of Africa. 2007;**18**(5):295-299

[75] Onwuchekwa AC, Ugwu EC. Pattern of rheumatic heart disease in adults in Maiduguri—North East Nigeria. Tropical Doctor. 1996;**26**(2):67-69

[76] Jaiyesimi F, Antia AU. Childhood rheumatic heart disease in Nigeria. Tropical and Geographical Medicine. 1981;**33**(1):8-13

[77] Jaiyesimi F, Antia AU. Prognostic factors in childhood rheumatic disease. Tropical and Geographical Medicine. 1981;**33**(1):14-38

[78] Fadahunsi HO, Coker AO, Usoro PD. Rheumatic heart disease in Nigerian children: Clinical and preventive aspects. Annals of Tropical Paediatrics. 1987;**7**(1):54-58

[79] Okoroma EO, Ihenacho IN, Anyanwu CH. Rheumatic fever in Nigerian children. A prospective study of 66 patients. American Journal of Diseases of Children. 1981; **135**(3):236-238

[80] Essop MR, Nkomo VT. Rheumatic and nonrheumatic valvular heart disease: Epidemiology, management, and prevention in Africa. Circulation. 2005;**112**(23):3584-3591

[81] Nkomo VT. Epidemiology and prevention of valvular heart diseases and infective endocarditis in Africa. Heart. 2007;**93**(12):1510-1519

[82] Nkomo VT et al. Burden of valvular heart diseases: A population-based study. Lancet. 2006;**368**(9540):1005-1011

[83] Cole TO, Adeleye JA. Rheumatic heart disease and pregnancy in Nigerian women. Clinical Cardiology. 1982;**5**(4):280-285

[84] Cole TO. Rheumatic fever and rheumatic heart disease in the tropics with particular reference to Nigeria. Nigerian Medical Journal. 1976;**6**(2):123-126

[85] Gunther G, Asmera J, Parry E. Death from rheumatic heart disease in rural Ethiopia. Lancet. 2006;**367**(9508):391

[86] Sliwa K et al. Incidence and characteristics of newly diagnosed rheumatic heart disease in urban African adults: Insights from the heart of Soweto study. European Heart Journal. 2009;**31**(6):719-727

[87] Falase AO, Sekoni GA, Adenle AD. Dilated cardiomyopathy in young adult Africans: A sequel to infections? African Journal of Medicine and Medical Sciences. 1982;**11**(1):1-5

[88] Falase AO, Fabiyi A, Ogunba EO. Heart muscle disease in Nigerian adults: A multifactorial disease. African Journal of Medicine and Medical Sciences. 1977;**6**(4):165-176

[89] Basile U et al. Thiamine deficiency and idiopathic cardiomegaly in Nigerian adults. A preliminary communication. The African Journal of Medical Sciences. 1973;**4**(4):465-469

[90] Falase AO. Heart muscle disease among adult Nigerians: Role of nutritional factors in its aetiology. European Journal of Cardiology. 1979;**10**(3):197-204

[91] Falase AO. Cardiomegaly of unknown origin among Nigerian adults: Role of hypertension in its aetiology. British Heart Journal. 1977;**39**(6):671-679

[92] Mayosi BM. Contemporary trends in the epidemiology and management of cardiomyopathy and pericarditis in sub-Saharan Africa. Heart. 2007;**93**(10):1176-1183

[93] Owor R, Rwomushana RJ. Familial congestive cardiomyopathy in Uganda. East African Medical Journal. 1975;**52**(7):372-375

[94] Przybojewski JZ et al. Familial dilated (congestive) cardiomyopathy. Occurrence in two brothers and an overview of the literature. South African Medical Journal. 1984;**66**(1): 26-30

[95] Maharaj B, Hammond MG. HLA-A, B, DR, and DQ antigens in black patients with idiopathic dilated cardiomyopathy. The American Journal of Cardiology. 1990;**65**(20): 1402-1403

[96] Maharaj B et al. HLA-A, B, DR, and DQ antigens in black patients with severe chronic rheumatic heart disease. Circulation. 1987;**76**(2):259-261

[97] Mayosi BM et al. Cardiac and skeletal actin gene mutations are not a common cause of dilated cardiomyopathy. Journal of Medical Genetics. 1999;**36**(10):796-797

[98] Sliwa K et al. Effects of pentoxifylline on cytokine profiles and left ventricular performance in patients with decompensated congestive heart failure secondary to idiopathic dilated cardiomyopathy. The American Journal of Cardiology. 2002;**90**(10):1118-1122

[99] Davies JN, Ball JD. The pathology of endomyocardial fibrosis in Uganda. British Heart Journal. 1955;**17**(3):337-359

[100] Davies JN. Endomyocardial fibrosis in Uganda. The Central African Journal of Medicine. 1956;**2**(9):323-328

[101] Davies JN. The ridge in endomyocardial fibrosis. Lancet. 1968;**1**(7543):631-632

[102] Hutt MSR et al. Cardiomyopathies. Bulletin of the World Health Organisation. 1965; **33**:257-288

[103] Shaper AG. Cardiovascular disease in the tropics. II. Endomyocardial fibrosis. British Medical Journal. 1972;**3**(5829):743-746

[104] Parry EH, Abrahams DG. The natural history of endomyocardial fibrosis. The Quarterly Journal of Medicine. 1965;**34**(136):383-408

[105] Mocumbi AO et al. A population study of endomyocardial fibrosis in a rural area of Mozambique. The New England Journal of Medicine. 2008;**359**(1):43-49

[106] Shaper AG. The geographical distribution of endomyocardial fibrosis. Pathology & Microbiology (Basel). 1970;**35**(1):26-35

[107] Adi FC. Endomyocardial fibrosis in two brothers. British Heart Journal. 1963;**25**:684-688

[108] Bukhman G, Ziegler J, Parry E. Endomyocardial fibrosis: Still a mystery after 60 years. PLoS Neglected Tropical Diseases. 2008;**2**(2):e97

[109] Ellis J et al. Echocardiographic, chest X-ray and electrocardiogram findings in children presenting with heart failure to a Ugandan paediatric ward. Tropical Doctor. 2007;**37**(3):149-150

[110] Akinwusi PO, Odeyemi AO. The changing pattern of endomyocardial fibrosis in South-West Nigeria. Clinical Medicine Insights: Cardiology. 2012;**6**:163-168

[111] Isezuo SA, Abubakar SA. Epidemiologic profile of peripartum cardiomyopathy in a tertiary care hospital. Ethnicity & Disease. 2007;**17**(2):228-233

[112] Sliwa K, Fett J, Elkayam U. Peripartum cardiomyopathy. Lancet. 2006;**368**(9536):687-693

[113] Ntusi NB, Mayosi BM. Aetiology and risk factors of peripartum cardiomyopathy: A systematic review. International Journal of Cardiology. 2009;**131**(2):168-179

[114] Abboud J et al. Peripartum cardiomyopathy: A comprehensive review. International Journal of Cardiology. 2007;**118**(3):295-303

[115] Tibazarwa K, Sliwa K. Peripartum cardiomyopathy in Africa: Challenges in diagnosis, prognosis, and therapy. Progress in Cardiovascular Diseases. 2010;**52**(4):317-325

[116] Isezuo SA et al. Case report: Acute limb ischaemia and gangrene associated with peripartum cardiomyopathy. The Nigerian Postgraduate Medical Journal. 2005; **12**(3):237-240

[117] Ramaraj R, Sorrell VL. Peripartum cardiomyopathy: Causes, diagnosis, and treatment. Cleveland Clinic Journal of Medicine. 2009;**76**(5):289-296

[118] Sliwa K et al. Current state of knowledge on aetiology, diagnosis, management, and therapy of peripartum cardiomyopathy: A position statement from the Heart Failure Association of the European Society of Cardiology Working Group on peripartum cardiomyopathy. European Journal of Heart Failure. 2010;**12**(8):767-778

[119] Adesanya CO et al. Peripartum cardiac failure. A ten year follow-up study. Tropical and Geographical Medicine. 1989;**41**(3):190-196

[120] Ford L et al. The outcome of peripartum cardiac failure in Zaria, Nigeria. QJM: An International Journal of Medicine. 1998;**91**(2):93-103

[121] Sliwa K et al. Evaluation of bromocriptine in the treatment of acute severe peripartum cardiomyopathy: A proof-of-concept pilot study. Circulation. 2010;**121**(13):1465-1473

[122] Lewis BS et al. Hypertrophic obstructive cardiomyopathy in the South African Bantu. South African Medical Journal. 1973;**47**(14):599-604

[123] Colyn HJ, Kleynhans PH. Hypertrophic cardiomyopathy in the black population of South Africa. South African Medical Journal. 1990;**77**(3):165

[124] Neutel JM, Myburgh DP. Apical hypertrophic nonobstructive cardiomyopathy in a pilot. Aviation, Space, and Environmental Medicine. 1987;**58**(10):1005-1008

[125] Myburgh DP et al. Apical hypertrophic cardiomyopathy. A case report. South African Medical Journal. 1987;**71**(6):392-393

[126] Przybojewski JZ, Blake RS. Hypertrophic non-obstructive apical cardiomyopathy. A case presentation and review of the literature. South African Medical Journal. 1984; **66**(13):492-498

[127] Lewis BS et al. Hypertrophic cardiomyopathy in South African blacks. South African Medical Journal. 1983;**63**(8):266-270

[128] Abegaz B. The impact of echocardiography in the diagnosis of hypertrophic cardiomyopathy. East African Medical Journal. 1990;**67**(8):556-567

[129] Posen BM et al. Clinical and prognostic evaluation of familial hypertrophic cardiomyopathy in two South African families with different cardiac beta myosin heavy chain gene mutations. British Heart Journal. 1995;**74**(1):40-46

[130] van der Merwe L et al. Genetic variation in angiotensin-converting enzyme 2 gene is associated with extent of left ventricular hypertrophy in hypertrophic cardiomyopathy. Human Genetics. 2008;**124**(1):57-61

[131] Heradien M et al. Race and gender representation of hypertrophic cardiomyopathy or long QT syndrome cases in a South African research setting. Cardiovascular Journal of Africa. 2007;**18**(5):312-315

[132] Moolman-Smook J et al. Identification of novel interactions between domains of myosin binding protein-C that are modulated by hypertrophic cardiomyopathy missense mutations. Circulation Research. 2002;**91**(8):704-711

[133] Blair E et al. Mutations of the light meromyosin domain of the beta-myosin heavy chain rod in hypertrophic cardiomyopathy. Circulation Research. 2002;**90**(3):263-269

[134] Andersen PS et al. Myosin light chain mutations in familial hypertrophic cardiomyopathy: Phenotypic presentation and frequency in Danish and South African populations. Journal of Medical Genetics. 2001;**38**(12):E43

[135] Moolman-Smook JC et al. Hypertrophic cardiomyopathy repealing tenets in South Africa. Cardiovascular Journal of South Africa. 2000;**11**(4):202-209

[136] Moolman-Smook JC et al. The origins of hypertrophic cardiomyopathy-causing mutations in two South African subpopulations: A unique profile of both independent and founder events. American Journal of Human Genetics. 1999;**65**(5):1308-1320

[137] Moolman-Smook JC et al. Identification of a new missense mutation in MyBP-C associated with hypertrophic cardiomyopathy. Journal of Medical Genetics. 1998;**35**(3):253-254

[138] Moolman JC, Brink PA, Corfield VA. Identification of a novel Ala797Thr mutation in exon 21 of the beta-myosin heavy chain gene in hypertrophic cardiomyopathy. Human Mutation. 1995;**6**(2):197-198

[139] Moolman JC, Brink PA, Corfield VA. Identification of a new missense mutation at Arg403, a CpG mutation hotspot, in exon 13 of the beta-myosin heavy chain gene in hypertrophic cardiomyopathy. Human Molecular Genetics. 1993;**2**(10):1731-1732

[140] Revera M et al. Long-Term Follow-Up of R403W MYH7 and R92W TNNT2 HCM Families: Mutations Determine Left Ventricular Dimensions but Not Wall Thickness during Disease Progression. 2007

[141] Revera M et al. Troponin T and β-myosin mutations have distinct cardiac functional effects in hypertrophic cardiomyopathy patients without hypertrophy. Cardiovascular Research. 2008;**77**(4):687-694

[142] Heradien M et al. Abnormal blood pressure response to exercise occurs more frequently in hypertrophic cardiomyopathy patients with the R92W troponin T mutation than in those with myosin mutations. Heart Rhythm. 2009;**6**(11):S18-S24

[143] Carstens N et al. Genetic variation in angiotensin II type 2 receptor gene influences extent of left ventricular hypertrophy in hypertrophic cardiomyopathy independent of blood pressure. Journal of the Renin-Angiotensin Aldosterone System. 2011;**12**(3):274-280

[144] Munclinger MJ, Patel JJ, Mitha AS. Follow-up of patients with arrhythmogenic right ventricular cardiomyopathy dysplasia. South African Medical Journal. 2000;**90**(1):61-68

[145] Matolweni LO et al. Arrhythmogenic right ventricular cardiomyopathy type 6 (ARVC6): Support for the locus assignment, narrowing of the critical region and mutation screening of three candidate genes. BMC Medical Genetics. 2006;**7**:29

[146] Watkins DA et al. Clinical features, survival experience, and profile of plakophylin-2 gene mutations in participants of the arrhythmogenic right ventricular cardiomyopathy registry of South Africa. Heart Rhythm. 2009;**6**(Suppl 11):S10-S17

[147] Hendricks N, Watkins DA, Mayosi BM. Lessons from the first report of the arrhythmogenic right ventricular cardiomyopathy registry of South Africa. Cardiovascular Journal of Africa. 2010;**21**(3):129-130

[148] Ker J, Van Der Merwe C. Isolated left ventricular non-compaction as a cause of thrombo-embolic stroke: A case report and review. Cardiovascular Journal of South Africa. 2006;**17**(3):146-147

[149] Massoure PL et al. Rare cause of heart failure in an elderly woman in Djibouti: Left ventricular non compaction. Medecine Tropicale (Mars). 2011;**71**(5):505-507

[150] Peters F et al. Isolated left ventricular noncompaction in sub-Saharan Africa: A clinical and echocardiographic perspective. Circulation. Cardiovascular Imaging. 2012; **5**(2):187-193

[151] Peters F et al. Isolated left ventricular noncompaction in identical twins. The American Journal of Cardiology. 2012;**110**(8):1175-1179

[152] Ali SK. Unique features of non-compaction of the ventricular myocardium in Arab and African patients. Cardiovascular Journal of Africa. 2008;**19**(5):241-245

[153] Ogah OS et al. Isolated left ventricular noncompaction: Report of a case from Ibadan, Nigeria. Nigerian Journal of Cardiology. 2016;**13**(2):148

[154] Sani MU et al. Human immunodeficiency virus (HIV) related heart disease: A review. Wiener Klinische Wochenschrift. 2005;**117**(3):73-81

[155] Syed FF, Sani MU. Recent advances in HIV-associated cardiovascular diseases in Africa. Heart. 2013;**99**(16):1146-1153

[156] Tukei VJ et al. Safety and tolerability of antiretroviral therapy among HIV-infected children and adolescents in Uganda. Journal of Acquired Immune Deficiency Syndromes. 2012;**59**(3):274-280

[157] Twagirumukiza M et al. Prevalence of dilated cardiomyopathy in HIV-infected African patients not receiving HAART: A multicenter, observational, prospective, cohort study in Rwanda. Current HIV Research. 2007;**5**(1):129-137

[158] Niakara A et al. Cardiovascular diseases and HIV infection: Study of 79 cases at the National Hospital of Ouagadougou (Burkina Faso). Bulletin de la Société de Pathologie Exotique. 2002;**95**(1):23-26

[159] Olusegun-Joseph DA et al. Echocardiographic patterns in treatment-naive HIV-positive patients in Lagos, South-West Nigeria. Cardiovascular Journal of Africa. 2012;**23**(8):e1-e6

[160] Sliwa K et al. Contribution of the human immunodeficiency virus/acquired immunodeficiency syndrome epidemic to de novo presentations of heart disease in the Heart of Soweto Study cohort. European Heart Journal. 2012;**33**(7):866-874

[161] Ladipo GO. Cardiac failure at Ahmadu Bello University Hospital, Zaria. Nigerian Medical Journal. 1978;**8**(2):96-99

[162] Bertrand E, Coulibaly AO, Ticolat R. Statistiques 1988, 1989 et 1990 de I'Institut de Cardiologie d' Abidjan. Cardiologie Tropicale. 1991;**17**(68):151-155

[163] Tantchou Tchoumi JC et al. Occurrence and pattern of congenital heart diseases in a rural area of sub-Saharan Africa. Cardiovascular Journal of Africa. 2011;**22**(2):63-66

[164] Marijon E et al. Prevalence of congenital heart disease in schoolchildren of sub-Saharan Africa, Mozambique. International Journal of Cardiology. 2006;**113**(3):440-441

[165] Sani MU, Mukhtar-Yola M, Karaye KM. Spectrum of congenital heart disease in a tropical environment: An echocardiography study. Journal of the National Medical Association. 2007;**99**(6):665-669

[166] Bassili A et al. Congenital heart disease among school children in Alexandria, Egypt: An overview on prevalence and relative frequencies. Journal of Tropical Pediatrics. 2000;**46**(6):357-362

[167] Bannerman CH, Mahalu W. Congenital heart disease in Zimbabwean children. Annals of Tropical Paediatrics. 1998;**18**(1):5-12

[168] Kokou O et al. The use of Doppler echocardiography in the diagnosis of congenital heart disease in the Pediatric Department of CHU-Tokoin, at Lome (Togo). Santé. 1996;**6**(3):161-164

[169] Jaiyesimi F, Antia AU. Congenital heart disease in Nigeria: A ten-year experience at UCH, Ibadan. Annals of Tropical Paediatrics. 1981;**1**(2):77-85

[170] McLaren MJ, Lachman AS, Barlow JB. Prevalence of congenital heart disease in black schoolchildren of Soweto, Johannesburg. British Heart Journal. 1979;**41**(5):554-558

[171] Antia AU. Congenital heart disease in Nigeria. Clinical and necropsy study of 260 cases. Archives of Disease in Childhood. 1974;**49**(1):36-39

[172] Levin SE, Kanarek KS. The incidence of congenital heart disease in Johannesburg. A 5-year study of liveborn infants at the Queen Victoria Maternity Hospital. South African Medical Journal. 1973;**47**(40):1855-1858

[173] van der Horst RL. The pattern and frequency of congenital heart disease among blacks. South African Medical Journal. 1985;**68**(6):375-378

[174] van der Horst, R.L. and J. Wainwright, Congenital heart disease in the Bantu: An autopsy analysis of 123 cases. South African Medical Journal. 1969;**43**(20): p. 586-589

[175] Wood JB, Serumaga J, Lewis MG. Congenital heart disease at necropsy in Uganda. A 16-years survey at Mulago Hospital, Kampala. British Heart Journal. 1969;**31**(1):76-79

[176] Gupta B, Antia AU. Incidence of congenital heart disease in Nigerian children. British Heart Journal. 1967;**29**(6):906-909

[177] Schrire V. Experience with congenital heart disease at Groote Schuur Hospital, Cape Town. An analysis of 1439 patients over an eleven-year period. South African Medical Journal. 1963;**37**:1175-1180

[178] Caddell JL, Morton P. The pattern of congenital heart disease in Yoruba children of Western Nigeria. American Heart Journal. 1967;**73**(3):431-432

[179] Caddell JL, Connor DH. Congenital heart disease in Ugandan children. British Heart Journal. 1966;**28**(6):766-767

[180] Williams AO. Coronary atherosclerosis in Nigeria. British Heart Journal. 1971;**33**(1):95-100

[181] Edington GM. Cardiovascular disease as a cause of death in the Gold Coast African. Transactions of the Royal Society of Tropical Medicine and Hygiene. 1954;**48**(5):419-425

[182] Falase AO, Cole TO, Osuntokun BO. Myocardial infarction in Nigerians. Tropical and Geographical Medicine. 1974;**25**(2):147-150

[183] Okuwobi BO. Pattern of heart diseases in Lagos. East African Medical Journal. 1968;**45**(3):122-127

[184] Bertrand E. Coronary heart disease in black Africans: An overview. East African Medical Journal. 1995;**72**(1):37-41

[185] Ikama MS et al. Heart failure in elderly patients in Brazzaville, Congo: Clinical and etiologic aspects and outcome. Medecine Tropicale (Mars). 2008;**68**(3):257-260

[186] Annual Report of Medical officer of Health. City of Johannesburg, Johannesburg. 1994

[187] Cosnett JE. Heart disease in the Zulu: Especially cardiomyopathy and cardiac infarction. British Heart Journal. 1962;**24**:76-82

[188] Schrire V. Heart disease in Southern Africa with special reference to ischaemic heart disease. South African Medical Journal. 1971;**45**(23):634-644

[189] Schwartz MB, Schamroth L, Seftel HC. The pattern of heart disease in the urbanized Johannesburg African. Medical Proceedings. 1958;**4**:275

[190] Sofowora EO. Pulmonary heart disease in Ibadan. Thorax. 1971;**26**(3):339-342

[191] Turner PP. Pulmonary heart disease in Africans in Mombasa. East African Medical Journal. 1962;**39**:40-51

[192] Okuwobi BO. Pattern of heart failure at Lagos University Teaching Hospital. The West African Medical Journal and Nigerian Practitioner. 1967;**16**(6):198-203

[193] Toure NO et al. Chronic cor pulmonale: A study of 34 cases in the Dakar University Hospital Center Cardiology Department. Dakar Médical. 2000;**45**(2):108-112

[194] Thienemann F et al. The causes, treatment, and outcome of pulmonary hypertension in Africa: Insights from the Pan African Pulmonary Hypertension cohort (PAPUCO) registry. International Journal of Cardiology. 2016;**221**:205-211

[195] Dzudie A et al. Pulmonary hypertension as seen in a rural area in sub-Saharan Africa: High prevalence, late clinical presentation and a high short-term mortality rate during follow up. Cardiovascular Journal of Africa. 2018;**29**(4):208-212

[196] Steenekamp JH, Simson IW, Theron W. Cardiovascular causes of death at Tshepong Hospital in 1 year, 1989-1990. A necropsy study. South African Medical Journal. 1992;**81**(3):142-146

[197] Hakim JG, Matenga JA, Siziya S. Myocardial dysfunction in human immunodeficiency virus infection: An echocardiographic study of 157 patients in hospital in Zimbabwe. Heart. 1996;**76**(2):161-165

[198] Aliyu ZY et al. Prevalence and risk factors for pulmonary artery systolic hypertension among sickle cell disease patients in Nigeria. American Journal of Hematology. 2008;**83**(6):485-490

[199] Diop IB et al. Congenital cardiopathies: Anatomo-clinical, prognostic, and therapeutic features apropos of 103 cases seen at the cardiology Clinic of the Dakar University Hospital Center. Dakar Médical. 1995;**40**(2):181-186

[200] Mpe MT. An uncommon cause of pulmonary hypertension. Cardiovascular Journal of South Africa. 2000;**11**(2):98-101

[201] Turner PP. Schistosomal pulmonary arterial hypertension in East Africa. British Heart Journal. 1964;**26**:821-831

[202] Grobbelaar J et al. Pulmonary hypertension due to recurrent juvenile laryngeal papillomatosis. International Journal of Pediatric Otorhinolaryngology. 2005;**69**(9):1279-1282

[203] Govender D, Pillay SV. Right pulmonary artery sarcoma. Pathology. 2001;**33**(2):243-245

[204] Heath D et al. A pulmonary hypertension-producing plant from Tanzania. Thorax. 1975;**30**(4):399-404

[205] Desai DK et al. Cardiac abnormalities in pulmonary oedema associated with hypertensive crises in pregnancy. British Journal of Obstetrics and Gynaecology. 1996; **103**(6):523-528

[206] McCulloch M et al. Angiographic features of 26 children with Takayasu's arteritis. Pediatric Radiology. 2003;**33**(4):230-235

[207] Bouldouyre M et al. Primary arterial pulmonary hypertension and sildenafil: A case report from Dakar. Dakar Médical. 2006;**51**(2):78-80

[208] Ansa VO et al. Seasonal variation in admission for heart failure, hypertension and stroke in Uyo, South-Eastern Nigeria. Annals of African Medicine. 2008;**7**(2):62-66

[209] Makubi A et al. Prevalence and prognostic implications of anaemia and iron deficiency in Tanzanian patients with heart failure. Heart. 2015;**101**(8):592-599

[210] Ojji D et al. A predominance of hypertensive heart failure in the Abuja Heart Study cohort of urban Nigerians: A prospective clinical registry of 1515 de novo cases. European Journal of Heart Failure. 2013;**15**(8):835-842

[211] Onwuchekwa AC, Asekomeh GE. Pattern of heart failure in a Nigerian teaching hospital. Vascular Health and Risk Management. 2009;**5**:745-750

[212] Familoni OB, Olunuga TO, Olufemi BW. A clinical study of pattern and factors affecting outcome in Nigerian patients with advanced heart failure. Cardiovascular Journal of Africa. 2007;**18**(5):308-311

[213] Owusu I. Causes of heart failure as seen in Kumasi, Ghana. Internet Journal of Third World Medicine. 2007;**5**:201-214

[214] Kingue S et al. A new look at adult chronic heart failure in Africa in the age of the Doppler echocardiography: Experience of the medicine department at Yaounde General Hospital. Annales de Cardiologie et d'Angeiologie. 2005;**54**(5):276-283

[215] Thiam M. Cardiac insufficiency in the African cardiology milieu. Bulletin de la Societe de Pathologie Exotique (1990). 2003;**96**(3):217-218

[216] Ogah OS et al. Gender differences in clinical characteristics and outcome of acute heart failure in sub-Saharan Africa: Results of the THESUS-HF study. Clinical Research in Cardiology. 2015;**104**(6):481-490

[217] Lee G et al. Are ECG abnormalities common in black Africans with heart failure? Results from the Heart of Soweto Study. SA Heart. 2008;**5**(1):4-11

[218] Dzudie A et al. Prognostic significance of ECG abnormalities for mortality risk in acute heart failure: Insight from the sub-Saharan Africa survey of heart failure (THESUS-HF). Journal of Cardiac Failure. 2014;**20**(1):45-52

[219] Sani MU et al. Echocardiographic predictors of outcome in acute heart failure patients in sub-Saharan Africa: Insights from THESUS-HF. Cardiovascular Journal of Africa. 2017;**28**(1):60-67

[220] Bonsu KO et al. Clinical characteristics and prognosis of patients admitted for heart failure: A 5-year retrospective study of African patients. International Journal of Cardiology. 2017;**238**:128-135

[221] Nyaga UF et al. Data on the epidemiology of heart failure in sub-Saharan Africa. Data in Brief. 2018;**17**:1218-1239

[222] Gallagher J et al. Heart failure in sub-Saharan Africa. Cardiac Failure Review. 2018; **4**(1):21-24

[223] Sani MU et al. Prevalence, clinical characteristics and outcomes of valvular atrial fibrillation in a cohort of African patients with acute heart failure: Insights from the THESUS-HF registry. Cardiovascular Journal of Africa. 2018;**29**(3):139-145

[224] Karaye KM, Sani MU. Factors associated with poor prognosis among patients admitted with heart failure in a Nigerian Tertiary Medical Centre: A cross-sectional study. BMC Cardiovascular Disorders. 2008;**8**:16

[225] Kuule JK, Seremba E, Freers J. Anaemia among patients with congestive cardiac failure in Uganda—Its impact on treatment outcomes. South African Medical Journal. 2009;**99**(12):876-880

[226] Ola BA et al. Relationship between depression and quality of life in Nigerian outpatients with heart failure. Journal of Psychosomatic Research. 2006;**61**(6):797-800

[227] Ansa VO et al. Psychological distress in Nigerian patients with heart failure. CVD Prevention and Control. 2009;**4**(4):207-211

[228] Mbakwem AC, Aina OF. Comparative study of depression in hospitalized and stable heart failure patients in an urban Nigerian teaching hospital. General Hospital Psychiatry. 2008;**30**(5):435-440

[229] Verena R et al. Medication adherence, self-care behaviour and knowledge on heart failure in urban South Africa: The heart of Soweto study. Cardiovascular Journal of Africa. 2010;**21**(2):86

[230] Bhagat K, Mazayi-Mupanemunda M. Compliance with medication in patients with heart failure in Zambabwe. East African Medical Journal. 2001;**78**(1):45-48

[231] Inglis SC et al. Anaemia and renal function in heart failure due to idiopathic dilated cardiomyopathy. European Journal of Heart Failure. 2007;**9**(4):384-390

[232] Dzudie A et al. Chronic heart failure, selected risk factors and co-morbidities among adults treated for hypertension in a cardiac referral hospital in Cameroon. European Journal of Heart Failure. 2008;**10**(4):367-372

[233] Tantchou TJ et al. Occurrence, aetiology and challenges in the management of congestive heart failure in sub-Saharan Africa: Experience of the Cardiac Centre in Shisong, Cameroon. Pan African Medical Journal. 2011;**8**:11(1):11-18

[234] Agbor VN et al. Heart failure in sub-Saharan Africa: A contemporaneous systematic review and meta-analysis. International Journal of Cardiology. 2018;**257**:207-215

[235] Mbakwem A et al. Comparative analysis of the quality of life of heart failure patients in South Western Nigeria. World Journal of Cardiovascular Diseases. 2013;**3**(1):146-153

[236] Kimani KN, Murray SA, Grant L. Spiritual issues of people living and dying with advanced heart failure in Kenya: A qualitative serial interview study. BMJ Global Health. 2016;**1**(3):e000077

[237] Cook C et al. The annual global economic burden of heart failure. International Journal of Cardiology. 2014;**171**(3):368-376

[238] Fonn S et al. 'Birth to Ten'—Pilot studies to test the feasibility of a birth cohort study investigating the effects of urbanisation in South Africa. South African Medical Journal. 1991;**79**(8):449-454

[239] Nieminen MS et al. EuroHeart failure survey II (EHFS II): A survey on hospitalized acute heart failure patients: Description of population. European Heart Journal. 2006;**27**(22):2725-2736

[240] Adams KF Jr et al. Characteristics and outcomes of patients hospitalized for heart failure in the United States: Rationale, design, and preliminary observations from the first 100,000 cases in the acute decompensated heart failure national registry (ADHERE). American Heart Journal. 2005;**149**(2):209-216

[241] Fonarow GC et al. Characteristics, treatments, and outcomes of patients with preserved systolic function hospitalized for heart failure: A report from the OPTIMIZE-HF registry. Journal of the American College of Cardiology. 2007;**50**(8):768-777

[242] Siswanto BB et al. Heart failure in NCVC Jakarta and 5 hospitals in Indonesia. CVD Prevention and Control. 2010;**5**:35-38

[243] Tsuchihashi-Makaya M et al. Characteristics and outcomes of hospitalized patients with heart failure and reduced vs. preserved ejection fraction. Report from the Japanese Cardiac Registry of Heart Failure in Cardiology (JCARE-CARD). Circulation Journal. 2009;**73**(10):1893-1900

Therapeutic Drug Monitoring of Micophenolate Mofetil in Cardiac Transplant Patients by Limited Sampling Strategy: An Update

Massimo Baraldo, Sandro Sponga and Ugolino Livi

Additional information is available at the end of the chapter

http://dx.doi.org/10.5772/intechopen.80027

Abstract

In the last few years, much progress in avoiding acute and chronic rejection in transplanted patients has been made by introducing new and more effective drugs with different formulations and combinations, and fewer side effects. Standardized protocols have been proposed for different organs, but individualized therapy based on immunosuppressive therapy blood monitoring is necessary because of pharmacological interaction, new generic drug introductions, and different absorptions and biodistributions. In specific mycophenolate mofetil dosing through mycophenolic acid (MPA), therapeutic drug monitoring has demonstrated minimal risk of organ transplant rejection. Even if the MPA area under the 12 h concentration–time curve is more accurate than MPA levels, it appears to be resource consuming and clinically impractical because of the need for numerous blood samples. Limited sampling strategy (LLS) has been proposed to overcome this problem. In heart-transplanted patients, MPA LSS is useful in guiding clinical management and dosing. The purpose of this chapter is to describe the state of the art of MPA LSS employment in heart transplantation and to perform an update of the scientific literature.

Keywords: heart transplantation, immunosuppressive therapy, mycophenolate mofetil, therapeutic drug monitoring, limited sampling strategy

1. Introduction

After heart transplantation, it is usual to administer the triple-drug therapy of induction and maintenance with calcineurin inhibitor (CNI), tacrolimus (TAC) or cyclosporine (CsA), mycophenolate mofetil (MMF)/enteric-coated mycophenolate sodium (EC-MPS), prodrugs of mycophenolic acid (MPA) or everolimus (EVE)/sirolimus (SIR) and corticosteroids (CSs). TAC should be the preferred CNI and MMF/EC-MPS the preferred cell cycle inhibitor [1]. Baraldo et al., in their review, concluded that CS withdrawal is safe in 50–80% of patients, with late withdrawal being better than early withdrawal. In addition, CS avoidance should be advisable and mandatory in pediatric patients, elderly patients and patients with insulin-dependent diabetes mellitus, metabolic disorders, osteoporosis and infections [2]. While for CNI or mTOR, therapeutic drug monitoring (TDM) is a clinical practice, MPA TDM is already controversial and is not widely used. One of the reasons is that in laboratories it was not a widely distributed platform for the analysis of plasma MPA concentrations, compared to other immunosuppressive drugs such as CsA, TAC, SIR and EVE. Moreover, this drug was promoted as not necessary for TDM and so generally MMF was administered as a fixed dose regimen. However, it was demonstrated that a >10-fold range in MPA dose-normalized area under the curve (AUC) between patients may be observed in heart, renal and liver transplantation, so MPA TDM may be useful [3]. Finally, since it has been demonstrated that the correct use of MPA TDM would require several blood samples to define the AUC_{0-12}, this approach appeared to be laborious, costly and clinically impractical [4]. To overcome the practical problems linked to blood samples to obtain an AUC_{0-12}, limited sampling strategies (LSSs) have been proposed. In a recent Consensus Meeting, LSSs were preferred in solid organ transplantation compared with drug dosing that is based on MPA through concentrations, and the individualization of MMF dosing may minimize the risk of organ transplant rejection [5]. So the MPA-AUC_{0-12} obtained using the LSS may be useful to guide clinical management and dosing. With the increasing use of MPA in solid organ transplantation, the greater possibility of analyzing at lower costs and the greater diffusion of laboratories that are able to perform the analysis have been recently revised for kidney transplantation [6]. The purpose of this chapter is to describe the state of the art of studies to calculate MPA LSSs in heart transplant recipients and to perform an update of the scientific literature.

2. Mycophenolate mofetil

MMF (Cell Cept®, Roche Pharmaceuticals, Basel, Switzerland) is the morpholino ester prodrug of MPA and was approved by the Food and Drug Administration in May 1995. MMF became a routine and extensively used part of immunosuppressive regimens, in combination with other immunosuppressant medications, after kidney transplantation, but it is also used after heart, lung, heart/lung and liver transplantation [7]. Attention was focused on the gastrointestinal side effects associated with its use, and an alternative formulation of MPA was explored in an effort to reduce the burden of gastrointestinal toxicity. An enteric-coated formulation of MPA (EC-MPS, Myfortic®, Novartis Pharma AG, Basel, Switzerland) was developed [8]. Equimolar doses of EC-MPS and MMF were shown to produce equivalent MPA exposure and to result in inhibition of the activity of the target enzyme inosine-5-monophosphate dehydrogenase (IMPDH) to a similar degree [9]. The patents have expired for MMF and EC-MPS. Because MPA is not considered a narrow therapeutic index drug, the wider bio-equivalence criteria are applied for the registration of generic MMF formulations [10].

2.1. Pharmacodynamics and pharmacokinetics

MMF is rapidly metabolized to its active constituent MPA, which acts as a specific inhibitor of the proliferation of T- and B-lymphocytes by reversibly inhibiting IMPDH, the key enzyme of the de novo purine synthesis in activated lymphocytes. The inhibition of T- and B-cell proliferation results in diminished cytotoxic T-cell responses and antibody formation against the allograft [11].

MPA bioavailability is >90%. It is mainly metabolized by uridine 5′-diphospho--glucuronosyltransferase [mycophenolic acid glucuronide (MPAG)] in the liver, intestine and kidney in 7-*O*-glucuronide (inactive) and acyl-glucuronide (active). MPA and MPAG are bound to the protein 97–99 and 82%, respectively, MPA metabolites are eliminated by the kidney and MPA and MPAG are subject to enterohepatic recirculation. The mean 'apparent' half-life and plasma clearance of MPA are 17.9 h and 11.6 L/h, respectively, after oral administration [12].

The clinical pharmacokinetics (PK) of MPA are characterized by a high between-subject and within-subject variability. It also was noted in all types of solid organ transplantation that dose-normalized MPA exposure in the first 3 months after transplantation was increased. The increase in MPA exposure can range from 30–80%. The coadministration of immunosuppressive or other drugs may influence MPA exposure. The MPA-AUC_{0-12} and its glucuronide metabolite were higher in patients with renal impairment than in patients with normal renal function following single dose administration. The MMF PK after a single dose is not altered in patients with cirrhosis. The main side effects of MPA are gastrointestinal disturbances, hematological disorders (e.g. anemia and leucopenia) and infections [13–15].

Moreover, it has been demonstrated that genetic polymorphisms may influence MMF absorption, distribution, metabolism and pharmacological action and may contribute to this interindividual variation in MMF response [16].

3. Mycophenolate mofetil after heart transplantations

Early preclinical studies of MMF demonstrated that MMF significantly prolonged cardiac transplants in rats and that the combination of MMF with CsA was more effective than either agent alone [17]. Furthermore, some trials suggest that MMF, when substituted for azathioprine in standard triple-drug therapy regimens, is well tolerated and might be more efficacious than azathioprine [18–20]. This could be explained by the hypothesis that MMF may provide more synergy with concomitantly administered cyclosporine and/or CSs than azathioprine, therefore demonstrating benefits to both renal [18–22] and cardiac transplant populations. Also, MMF has novel properties that may contribute to the prevention of cardiac allograft rejection and provide benefits in reducing the progression of vascular allograft vasculopathy (CAV).

3.1. Drug administration

Some findings have attempted to correlate MMF pharmacokinetic parameters with outcomes. MMF is a prodrug, so it is rapidly hydrolysed after ingestion to MPA. It must be administered on an empty stomach. TDM in patients receiving MMF has not been extensively investigated, although preclinical studies demonstrated a correlation between MPA levels and histologic severity of graft rejection. In addition, because appreciable within-patient fluctuations may occur, the dose should not be changed based on a single predose measurement. Another important point is the balance between the different immunosuppressive agents. For example, in previous studies, the risk of rejection was similar between groups with either a higher CsA level and a lower MMF dose or a lower CsA level and a higher MMF dose [23].

3.2. Trials supporting MMF

In 1993, Ensley et al. [18] published one of the first clinical reports describing the use of MMF in cardiac transplantation. This was the first study that found MMF effective to significantly reduce the mean biopsy score with less myelosuppression compared to azathioprine. Some years later, Kobashigawa et al. [24] published the first large multicentre trial in 1998. At the time the trial was initiated, immunosuppressive regimens for heart transplantation relied on a combination of CsA, steroids and azathioprine. The use of MMF demonstrated better survival rates at 1 and 5 years. After these promising results, an analysis of data from the Joint ISHLT/United Network for Organ Sharing Thoracic Registry was conducted in 2001 [25] where the improved long-term survival benefit of MMF therapy was confirmed, suggesting that the positive findings are broadly applicable within the cardiac transplant population. In addition to the randomized, multicentre trials [26–28], other trials and studies evaluated MMF in cardiac transplant recipients in combination with either CsA [29–32] or TAC [30] and in CNI-sparing regimens [33–35]. For example, other studies evaluating the combination of MMF with TAC were published, aimed at determining whether trough-level-adjusted MMF was more effective in combination with TAC or CsA. These results showed that the incidence of acute rejections was lower in patients receiving TAC versus the CsA group, although there was no difference in patient survival. Results from the most recent multicentre, randomized trial involving MMF in cardiac transplant recipients were presented at the ISHLT annual meeting in 2005 [36]. Hence, these authors concluded that in cardiac transplant patients, TAC/MMF appears to offer advantages over TAC/SRL or CsA/MMF when considering any treated rejection and side-effect profiles.

3.3. Advantages and side effects of MMF therapy

Therapy with MMF has peculiar advantages. In patients with chronic renal dysfunction, the reduction in CNI exposure, either through dose reduction or complete withdrawal, has been studied as a means of minimizing further deterioration of renal function. For this purpose, MMF-based CNI-sparing strategies were evaluated in three trials with promising results [34, 35, 37]. A second aspect is related to the anti-inflammatory properties of MMF that may provide long-term benefits in reducing the risk of CAV in cardiac transplant recipients. Furthermore, Weis et al. [37] reported that in cardiac transplant patients the combination of TAC/MMF appeared to be superior to TAC/azathioprine in preserving early coronary vasomotor function, endothelial nitric oxide synthase expression and inducible nitric oxide synthase suppression, as well as cardiac interleukin-6 release. Since these factors, in addition to the risks posed by rejection, are believed to be predictors of CAV, MMF may have a beneficial impact on the subsequent development of CAV.

Being a selective inhibitor of inosine monophosphate dehydrogenase, it is common to have some side effects. The most commonly reported side effects of MMF include leukopenia, anemia, infections, systemic cytomegalovirus disease, hypercholesterolemia and gastrointestinal complications such as diarrhea, nausea and dyspepsia. On the other hand, malignant neoplasms, especially of the skin, are frequent in patients treated with MMF [38, 39].

4. Therapeutic drug monitoring of MPA

Several studies have suggested that therapeutic drug monitoring of MPA concentrations in patients with renal, heart or lung transplants may improve clinical outcomes and allow effective dose individualization of MMF potentially minimizing toxicity [3, 40–43]. In heart transplant recipients, several studies have shown that MPA levels correlate to the risk of rejection [44, 45]. AUC_{0-12} seems to be a better parameter to optimize MPA treatment than the predose measurement (C_0). Unfortunately, measuring AUC_{0-12} requires the collection and analysis of multiple blood samples, which is costly and time-consuming for patients and clinical staff. So, AUC_{0-12} measurement could be simplified by using a technique, initially developed for anticancer drugs, called LSS [46, 47]. It was shown that an equation using three blood samples measured at specific times could approximate or estimate the real AUC_{0-12}. An AUC_{0-12} threshold of 50 mg × h/L was proposed (sensitivity = 77%, specificity = 25%) beyond which the risk of rejection was significantly increased (low vs. high: HR = 3.48 [1.21–10.0], $p = 0.0204$) [48].

4.1. Analysis of MPA

Quantification of MPA may be performed by high-performance liquid chromatography (HPLC) with ultraviolet detection, liquid chromatography-mass spectrometry (LC–MS/MS) or a commercially available platform assay. In general, laboratories that are providing a routine TDM service will tend to use the platform immunoassay. Those with a large number of sample loads and those with research interests are likely to use the chromatographic technique. HPLC with MS detection is often described as the gold standard technique [49, 50]. One of the problems that can create a bias and alter the calculation of the nomograms are the analytical methods used. It has now been demonstrated that MPA plasma concentrations measured by the immunoassay technique are higher than those determined by HPLC by 25–36%. This overestimation is most likely attributable to the cross-reactivity of the pharmacologically active acyl-glucoronide (Ac MPAG).

4.2. Limited sampling strategy

LSS is a technique aimed at estimating the AUC_{0-12} using a small number of samples, usually three or fewer. Modeling the relationship between the pharmacokinetic parameter and the drug concentration at various times allows this reduction in the number of samples required. The model can then be used to choose the best sampling times to determine the parameter accurately and precisely. The development of such a method requires full pharmacokinetic profiles drawn with sufficient points to measure AUC_{0-12} accurately. Most authors use the trapezoidal method, but there is also linear trapezoidal and linear-logarithmic trapezoidal.

The differences observed between methods are small and there is no clinical significance. To develop an LSS, the first step is arbitrarily splitting the patient data into two groups: a *training group* and a *testing* or *validation group*. The training group is used to determine the relationship between AUC_{0-12} and the timed blood concentration data using a linear regression. The AUC_{0-12} is considered to be the dependent variable; the independent variables are the blood concentrations at each time point. An equation is defined giving the AUC_{0-12} as a function of one or several concentrations:

$$AUC_{0-12} = \text{Constant} + (M_1 \times C_1) + (M_2 \times C_2) + (M_3 \times C_3) + (M_x \times C_x)$$

where AUC_{0-12} is the predicted AUC_{0-12}, constant is the intercept on the y-axis, C_1, C_2, C_3, C_x are the blood concentrations measured at time 1, 2, 3, x and M_1, M_2, M_3, M_x are the associated coefficients. The equations are then validated using the testing group. Validation is a compulsory step that must be carried out on a different group to the training group because testing an equation on the group of patients used to generate the equation itself would be self-fulfilling and therefore would produce biased results. Using a fresh data set allows the equations to be tested under real conditions, thus helping in the decision about which equations should be used and which should not. The performance of the equations can be assessed by comparing the *predicted* AUC_{0-12} with the *measured* AUC_{0-12} measuring the mean prediction error or bias (*me*) and the root mean squared prediction error or precision (*rmse*) with their confidence intervals (CIs). The smaller these parameters, the better the prediction [51]. A simpler assessment of the performance of the equations can be achieved by estimating the percentage prediction error (%pe) on the AUC_{0-12}, defined as ([predicted value − measured value]/measured value) times 100. A more clinically orientated method consists of evaluating the proportion of AUC_{0-12} estimated within a percentage prediction error range. Another method consists of expressing the results using the absolute prediction error for a certain percentile of predictions. Some authors 'validated' their equations by calculating the correlation coefficient (*r*) or coefficient of determination (*r*) between the predicted AUC_{0-12} and the measured AUC_{0-12}. This method should not be used because it gives biased results [52].

5. Limited sampling strategy in heart transplants: an upgrade

A search of MEDLINE was done for papers on heart transplantation, MPA and LSS. The following search terms were used: mycophenolic acid, mycophenolate mofetil, heart transplant, solid organ transplant and limited sampling strategy. We utilized this filter: human, adult and English. We considered only papers with these inclusion criteria: age > 18 years, heart transplantation, cotreatment with CyA or TAC and CSs, heart-training group, heart-testing group and plasma MPA concentrations analysed by HPLC. We excluded papers with: age < 18 years, kidney, lung, liver, pancreas transplantations and plasma MPA concentrations analysed by enzyme-multiplied immunoassay technique (EMIT). We found only five studies published, presented in **Table 1**, where we reported studies with the same analytical assay (HPLC) and the nomogram with a coefficient of determination $r^2 > 0.80$.

http://dx.doi.org/10.5772/intechopen.80027

No. of patients	Model equations AUC_{0-12} =	r^2	Method of analysis	Time of AUC; other drugs	Method used	References
9	5.57 + 0.90 * C1.25 + 2.02 * C2 + 4.59 * C6	0.93	HPLC	5 months; CsA, steroids	Training set	[53]
	3.8 + 1.03 * C1.25 + 1.82 * C2 + 1.57 * C4 + 3.48 * C6	0.95				
29	5.57 + 0.90 * C1.25 + 2.02 * C2 + 4.59 * C6	0.87			Validation set	[54]
	3.8 + 1.03 * C1.25 + 1.82 * C2 + 1.57 * C4 + 3.48* C6	0.81				
11	0.10 + 11.15 * C0 + 0.42 * C1 + 2.80 * C2	0.96	HPLC	9 months; CsA, steroids	Training set	[55]
	1.28 + 1.91 * C1 + 0.26 * C2 + 5.91 * C4	0.95				
	−0.51 + 11.47 * C0 + 3.24 * C2	0.94				
	−0.23 + 12.70 * C0 + 3.36 * C2–0.80 * C4	0.94				
28	1.25 * C1 + 5.29 * C4 + 2.90 * C8 + 3.61 * C10	0.95	HPLC	>6 months; TAC	Training set	[56]
	1.33 * C1 + 3.99 * C4 + 3.23 * C6 + 3.81 * C8	0.94				
	1.53 * C1 + 5.51 * C4 + 4.62 * C8	0.91				
	3.93 * C1 + 3.99 * C4 + 3.23 * C6 + 3.81 * C8	0.90				
	3.37 * C0 + 0.97 * C0.5 + 1.20 * C1 + 2.70 * C2	0.87				
	1.11 * C0.5 + 1.16 * C1 + 3.72 * C2	0.84				
20	$9.69 + 0.63 * C_{0.5} + 0.61 * C_1 + 2.20 * C_2$	0.84	HPLC	1–12 months; CsA, steroids	Training set	[57]
24	$7.93 + 3.89 * C_0 + 0.87 * C_1 + 1.02 * C_2 + 3.72 * C_4$	0.89			Validation set	
	$10.2 + 0.64 * C_1 + 0.62 * C_{1.5} + 3.03 * C_4 + 4.23 * C_6$	0.85				

AUC = area under the curve; r^2 = coefficient of determination; CsA = cyclosporine; HPLC = high-performance liquid chromatography; TAC = tacrolimus.

Table 1. Limited sampling strategy suggested for MPA-AUC monitoring in combination with cyclosporine A or tacrolimus in heart transplantation.

In 2005, Baraldo et al. wrote the first paper on the use of LSSs to estimate the AUC in heart transplant patients. This was one of two papers that utilized correctly training group and validation group. The authors studied a population with these characteristics: adult >18 years, Caucasian ethnicity, heart transplanted, first 3 months from transplantation, cotreated with

CsA and steroids and good kidney and liver functions. The analysis of MPA plasma concentrations was by HPLC. Multiple stepwise regression analysis was used to define the time points of MPA levels to explain the MPA-$AUC_{0–12}$. Agreement between abbreviated $AUC_{0–12}$ and full $AUC_{0–12}$ was tested by means of a Bland and Altman analysis. Stepwise linear regression showed that the minimal model with the best estimation of MPA-$AUC_{0–12}$ was obtained at time values of 1.25, 2 and 6 h. The corresponding estimated model was $AUC_{0–12} = 5.568 + 0.902 * C(1.25) + 2.022 * C(2) + 4.594 * C(6)$ ($r^2 = 0.926$). Bland and Altman analysis revealed good agreement between predicted $AUC_{0–12}$ and full $AUC_{0–12}$. A further interesting model equation obtained by four samples was $AUC_{0–12} = 3.800 + 1.015 * C(1.25) + 1.819 * C(2) + 1.566 * C(4) + 3.479 * C(6)$ ($r^2 = 0.948$) [53]. To obtain the validation, these two algorithms proposed were tested in a validation group (29 heart transplant recipients) with the same characteristics of the testing group. The two LSS algorithms used predicted the corresponding MPA-$AUC_{0–12}$ with a mean bias of −4.85 and −3.6% and mean precision of 15.9 and 14%, respectively. Baraldo et al. in conclusion revealed that the MPA-$AUC_{0–12}$ obtained using the LSS may be useful to guide clinical management and dosing, but in heart transplant recipients who share the same characteristics [54].

The study of Wada et al. published in 2007 studied 22 Japanese heart transplant patients approximately 9 months after transplantation and divided them into two groups: 11 who were given MMF + CsA and 11 who were given MMF + TAC. They calculated the entire MPA-$AUC_{0–12}$ and developed an LSS. They suggested a model consisting of three time points and another with two time points that predicted the entire MPA-$AUC_{0–12}$. We have utilized these two algorithms in heart transplant patients treated with MMF-CsA. The results obtained from this study, however, should be taken with caution because of the limited number of patients evaluated and the ethnic difference, which could influence MPA pharmacokinetics. The patients studied were given the same regimen therapy, the analytical method used was HPLC and the same pharmacokinetic and statistical approaches were used [55].

In 2008, Kaczmarek et al. studied 28 heart transplant patients treated with MMF and TAC. For each patient, the entire MPA-$AUC_{0–12}$ was studied using an LSS. The best estimation of MPA-$AUC_{0–12}$ was obtained with four sampling points: $AUC = 1.25 * C_1 + 5.29 * C_4 + 2.90 * C_8 + 3.61 * C_{10}$ ($r^2 = 0.95$). The three sampling point equation within the first 2 h was preferred for ambulatory patients: $AUC = 1.1 * C_{0.5} + 1.16 * C_1 + 3.72 * C_2$ ($r^2 = 0.84$). The population studied was long-term adult heart transplant recipients (2.5 ± 3 years) with chronic maintenance of immunosuppressive therapy consisting of MMF and TAC [56].

The most recent publication that defined algorithms for the TDM of MPA in heart transplant patients was by Pawinski et al. [57]. The authors studied 20 patients in a first step to obtain a *sampling strategy* and 24 patients in a second step to validate the algorithms. The regression equation for AUC estimation that gave the best fit was: $AUC = 9.69 + 0.63 * C_{0.5} + 0.61 * C_1 + 2.20 * C_2$ ($r^2 = 0.841$; *me* = 3.2%; CI 95% (−42.2%; 40.3%)). This global approach appears correct. However, there are some issues that must be discussed: (1) from a statistical point of view, the CI of the *me* is quite wide; (2) the authors calculated the algorithms within the range of 6–8 weeks to 1 year after heart transplant and validated the algorithms in patients more than 1 year after heart transplant, periods that might be characterized by different pathophysiological conditions and concomitant therapy; and (3) the algorithms that include the C_6 blood sample presented the same $r^2 = 0.841$ and should be considered [58].

Moreover, the study by Dosch et al. presented single-centre preliminary analysis data and is one of the largest published investigations of MPA-AUC_{0-12} in heart transplant recipients to date. The authors, however, did not calculate the entire AUC_{0-12}, and used algorithms taken from the literature with algorithms calculated in renal-transplanted patients. Furthermore, MPA plasma concentrations were measured by means of Emit Mycophenolic Acid Assay, which gives slightly higher concentration results compared to HPLC [59].

Ting et al. evaluated 25 heart transplant patients and estimated the MPA-AUC_{0-12}. They used an LSS previously developed for lung transplant recipients as well as an LSS used for heart transplant patients published from a different author. The authors concluded that the previously developed LSS used for lung transplant recipients performed well when applied to the heart transplant population for the prediction of MPA-AUC, while the application of the LSS obtained from the literature yielded fewer optimal results. Their conclusion was that: (1) LSS appears to be centre specific, (2) LSS should always be validated before implementation and (3) LSS should be limited to the population and drug therapy that were used to develop it [60].

6. Conclusions

This update has highlighted that research on MPA TDM by LSS in heart-transplanted patients was exhausted in 2009. Over the last 10 years, prevalent MPA TDM by LSS studies have been developed in kidney transplants and revised by van Gelder [6]. From the last Consensus Report, MPA TDM based on LSSs is preferred in solid organ transplantation compared to drug dosing that is based on single MPA trough concentrations. LSS is associated with early postoperative efficacy. The data suggest that specific patient populations might benefit from LSSs to reduce immunological risk in patients who are undergoing minimization or withdrawal of immunosuppressive therapy and patients who are experiencing altered renal, hepatic or bowel function [5]. Even though there is scientific support of its importance, the analysis of MPA plasma concentrations, LLS or Bayesian methodologies is not currently applied on a routine basis after heart transplant, and studies from heart transplant patients remain limited [53–57].

The most recent publication that defined algorithms for the TDM of MPA in heart transplant patients was by Pawinski et al. [57]. The authors calculated the algorithms within the range of 6–8 weeks to 1 year after heart transplant and validated the algorithms in patients more than 1 year after heart transplant. The two periods cannot be compared because the former is more or less rich in clinical problems and drugs, while the latter is usually characterized by a clinical stationarity and fewer medications taken.

Kaczmarek et al. studied 28 heart transplant patients treated with MMF and TAC [56]; the population studied was long-term adult heart transplant recipients (2.5 ± 3 years). These algorithms cannot be compared with MMF-CyA. An algorithm calculated from a TAC + MPA association cannot be used for a CsA + MPA association.

The study of Wada et al. considered patients with the same regimen therapy, analytical method (HPLC) and pharmacokinetic and statistical approaches [55]. In this study the approach appears well designed; however, ethnic differences could influence MPA pharmacokinetics, create a bias and generate nomograms that cannot be used for other ethnic groups. It appears that with the same dosage, MPA systemic exposure is higher in Asian renal transplant patients than in Caucasians and American-Africans [61].

Papers by Baraldo et al., ideation groups 2005 and validation groups 2009 are the only studies performed in the first 6 months after transplantation, which are the months where the greatest variability is observed and are the most critical months for the graft [53, 54]. In the Consensus of 2010, the group of experts cited the Kaczmarek, Baraldo and Ting papers, predicting them as reference works for the algorithms in heart transplants. One of the limitations of this study was the limited number of patients in the ideation group [5].

When using the LSS to estimate the MPA-AUC, it is important that the study populations (ideation group and validation group), the drugs and the analytical methods used have characteristics that are always the same and repeatable. Bayesian methodologies have multiple advantages, are more adaptable to different types of patients and are less sensitive to inaccuracies in sampling time [4, 62]. As a result the application of a nomogram from an LSS to estimate $AUC_{0–12}$ is simpler to use but requires greater precision, while Bayesian methodologies are more difficult to use and a specialized technician is required.

Thanks to research done on kidney transplants, today there are automated LC–MS/MS platforms on the market that can perform MPA plasma analysis more accurately, in less time and the costs of the analyses have been significantly reduced. Therefore, there is currently a greater possibility of performing the MPA TDM and a personalization of the therapy.

More accurate MPA TDM may reduce the leukopenia that often leads to discontinuation of MMF therapy and increased risk of rejection. Therefore, in heart transplantations it may be concluded that: (1) the guidelines recommend a C_0 of 1–3.5 mg/L and MPA-$AUC_{0–12}$ values of 30–60 mg · h/L; (2) a population is used similar to that for the calculation of the nomogram (type of transplant, post-transplant period, used therapy, ethnicity, etc.); and (3) analysis of the MPA is performed with a method similar to that used to calculate the nomogram of the LSS.

In conclusion, these results are interesting because LSS MPA-$AUC_{0–12}$ in heart transplant patients remains a sector of clinical pharmacology seldom studied and completes our previous findings with a validation group showing valuable bias and precision values. Future studies are needed to determine whether these algorithms can be clinically applied in a larger cohort of heart transplant patients receiving CsA or TAC associated with MPA therapy.

Acknowledgements

The authors thank the healthcare staff involved for the collection of blood samples and for the analyses performed.

No (external) funding was obtained for the writing this chapter.

http://dx.doi.org/10.5772/intechopen.80027

Conflict of interest

The authors have no conflicts of interest.

Author details

Massimo Baraldo[1,2,*], Sandro Sponga[4] and Ugolino Livi[3,4]

*Address all correspondence to: massimo.baraldo@uniud.it

1 Clinical Pharmacology, Department of Medical Area (DAME), University of Udine, Italy

2 SOC of Clinical Pharmacology and Toxicology Institute, University Hospital of Udine, Italy

3 Cardiac Surgery, Department of Medical Area (DAME), University of Udine, Italy

4 Cardiothoracic Department, University Hospital of Udine, Italy

References

[1] Söderlund C, Rådegran G. Immunosuppressive therapies after heart transplantation--The balance between under- and over- immunosuppression. Transplantation Review. 2015;**29**:181-189

[2] Baraldo M, Gregoraci G, Livi U. Steroid-free and steroid withdrawal protocols in heart transplantation: The review of literature. Transplant International. 2014;**27**:515-529

[3] Shaw LM, Koreka M, Venkataramanan R, et al. Mycophenolate acid pharmacodynamic and pharmacokinetic provide a basis for rational monitoring strategies. American Journal of Transplantation. 2003;**3**:534-542

[4] van Gelder TM, Le Meur YM, Shaw LM, et al. Therapeutic drug monitoring of mycophenolate mofetil in transplantation. Therapeutic Drug Monitoring. 2006;**28**:145-154

[5] Kuypers Dirk RJ, Le Meur Y, Cantarovich M, et al. Consensus report on therapeutic drug monitoring of mycophenolic acid in solid organ transplantation. Clinical Journal of the American Society of Nephrology. 2010;**5**:341-358

[6] van Gelder T et al. Mycophenolate revisited. Transplant International. 2015;**28**:508-515

[7] Opelz G, Döhler B, Süsal C. Analysis of positive kidney, heart, and liver transplant crossmatches reported to the Collaborative Transplant Study. Human Immunology. 2009;**70**:627-630

[8] Kaplan B. Enteric-coated mycophenolate sodium (Myfortic): An overview of current and future use in transplantation. Drugs. 2006;**66**(Suppl. 2):1-8

[9] Budde K, Bauer S, Hambach P, et al. Pharmacokinetic and pharmacodynamic comparison of enteric-coated mycophenolate sodium and mycophenolate mofetil in maintenance renal transplant patients. American Journal of Transplantation. 2007;**7**:888-898

[10] van Gelder T, Gabardi S. Method, strengths, weaknesses, and limitation of bioequivalence tests with special regard to immunosuppressive drugs. Transplant International. 2013;**26**:771-777

[11] Staatz CE, Tett SE. Clinical pharmacokinetics and pharmacodynamics of mycophenolate in solid organ transplant recipients. Clinical Pharmacokinetics. 2007;**46**:13-58

[12] Bulligaham R et al. Clinical pharmacokinetics of mycophenolate mofetil. Clinical Pharmacokinetics. 1998;**64**:429-455

[13] van Gelder T, Hilbrands LB, Vanrenterghem Y, et al. A randomized double-blind, multicenter plasma concentration controlled study of the safety and efficacy of oral mycophenolate mofetil for the prevention of acute rejection after kidney transplantation. Transplantation. 1999;**68**:261-266

[14] Le Meur Y, Buchler M, Thierry A, et al. Individualized mycophenolate mofetil dosing based on drug exposure significantly improves patient outcomes after renal transplantation. American Journal of Transplantation. 2007;**7**:2496-2503

[15] Gaston RS, Kaplan B, Shah T, et al. Fixed- or controlled-dose mycophenolate mofetil with standard- or reduced-dose calcineurin inhibitors: The Opticept trial. American Journal of Transplantation. 2009;**9**:1607-1619

[16] Hesselink DA, van Gelder T. Genetic and nongenetic determinants of between-patient variability in the pharmacokinetics of mycophenolic acid. Clinical Pharmacology and Therapeutics. 2005;**78**:317-321

[17] Morris RE, Hoyt EG, Murphy MP, et al. Mycophenolic acid morpholinoethyl ester (RS-61443) is a new immunosuppressant that prevents and halts heart allograft rejection by selective inhibition of T- and B-cell purine synthesis. Transplantation Proceedings. 1990;**22**:1659-1662

[18] Ensley RD, Bristow MR, Olsen SL, et al. The use of mycophenolate mofetil (RS-61443) in human heart transplant recipients. Transplantation. 1993;**56**:75-82

[19] Taylor DO, Ensley RD, Olsen SL, Dunn D, Renlund DG. Mycophenolate mofetil (RS-61443): Preclinical, clinical, and three-year experience in heart transplantation. The Journal of Heart and Lung Transplantation. 1994;**13**:571-582

[20] Renlund DG, Gopinathan SK, Kfoury AG, Taylor DO. Mycophenolate mofetil (MMF) in heart transplantation: Rejection prevention and treatment. Clinical Transplantation. 1996;**10**:136-139

[21] Sollinger HW. Mycophenolate mofetil for the prevention of acute rejection in primary cadaveric renal allograft recipients. Transplantation. 1995;**60**:225-232

[22] European Mycophenolate Mofetil Cooperative Study Group. Placebo-controlled study of mycophenolate mofetil combined with cyclosporin and corticosteroids for prevention of acute rejection. Lancet. 1995;**345**:1321-1325

[23] Cantarovich M, Giannetti N, Cecere R. Impact of cyclosporine 2-h level and mycophenolate mofetil dose on clinical outcomes in de novo heart transplant patients receiving anti-thymocyte globulin induction. Clinical Transplantation. 2003;**17**:144-150

[24] Kobashigawa J, Miller L, Renlund D, et al. A randomized active-controlled trial of mycophenolate mofetil in heart transplant recipients. Mycophenolate Mofetil Investigators. Transplantation. 1998;**66**:507-515

[25] Hosenpud JD, Bennett LE. Mycophenolate mofetil versus azathioprine in patients surviving the initial cardiac transplant hospitalization: An analysis of the Joint UNOS/ISHLT Thoracic Registry. Transplantation. 2001;**72**:1662-1665

[26] Hosenpud JD, Novick RJ, Bennett LE, et al. The Registry of the International Society for Heart and Lung Transplantation: Thirteenth Official Report—1996. The Journal of Heart and Lung Transplantation. 1996;**15**:655-674

[27] Miller LW, Naftel DC, Bourge RC, et al. Infection after heart transplantation: A multi-institutional study. Cardiac Transplant Research Database Group. The Journal of Heart and Lung Transplantation. 1994;**13**:381-392

[28] Eisen HJ, Kobashigawa J, Keogh A, et al. Three-year results of a randomized, double-blind, controlled trial of mycophenolate mofetil versus azathioprine in cardiac transplant recipients. The Journal of Heart and Lung Transplantation. 2005;**24**:517-525

[29] Meiser BM, Groetzner J, Kaczmarek I, et al. Tacrolimus or cyclosporine: Which is the better partner for mycophenolate mofetil in heart transplant recipients? Transplantation. 2004;**78**:591-598

[30] Taylor DO, Sharma RC, Kfoury AG, Renlund DG. Increased incidence of allograft rejection in stable heart transplant recipients after late conversion from mycophenolate mofetil to azathioprine. Clinical Transplantation. 1999;**13**:296-299

[31] Pethig K, Heublein B, Wahlers T, et al. Mycophenolate mofetil for secondary prevention of cardiac allograft vasculopathy: Influence on inflammation and progression of intimal hyperplasia. The Journal of Heart and Lung Transplantation. 2004;**23**:61-66

[32] Weigel G, Griesmacher A, Karimi A, et al. Effect of mycophenolate mofetil therapy on lymphocyte activation in heart transplant recipients. The Journal of Heart and Lung Transplantation. 2002;**21**:1074-1079

[33] Angermann CE, Stork S, Costard-Jackle A, et al. Reduction of cyclosporine after introduction of mycophenolate mofetil improves chronic renal dysfunction in heart transplant recipients—The IMPROVED multi-centre study. European Heart Journal. 2004;**25**:1626-1634

[34] Groetzner J, Meiser B, Landwehr P, et al. Mycophenolate mofetil and sirolimus as calcineurin inhibitor-free immunosuppression for late cardiac-transplant recipients with chronic renal failure. Transplantation. 2004;**77**:568-574

[35] Tedoriya T, Keogh AM, Kusano K, et al. Reversal of chronic cyclosporine nephrotoxicity after heart transplantation—Potential role of mycophenolate mofetil. The Journal of Heart and Lung Transplantation. 2002;**21**:976-982

[36] Kobashigawa J, Miller LW, Felker GM, et al. 12 month report of a 3 arm multicenter comparison of tacrolimus (TAC), MMF or TAC/sirolimus (SRL) and steroids vs cyclosporine microemulsion (CyA), MMF and steroids in de novo cardiac transplant recipients. The Journal of Heart and Lung Transplantation. 2005;**24**:S61-S62

[37] Weis M, Wildhirt SM, Schulze C, et al. Coronary vasomotor dysfunction in the cardiac allograft: Impact of different immunosuppressive regimens. Journal of Cardiovascular Pharmacology. 2000;**36**:776-784

[38] Miller LW, Naftel DC, Bourge RC, et al. Infection after heart transplantation: A multi-institutional study. The Journal of Heart and Lung Transplantation. 1994;**13**:381-392

[39] Kobashigawa JA, Katznelson S, Laks H, et al. Effect of pravastatin on outcomes after cardiac transplantation. The New England Journal of Medicine. 1995;**333**:621-627

[40] Dubrey SW, Holt DW, Banner N. Measurement of mycophenolate mofetil plasma levels after heart transplantation and a potential side effects of high levels. Therapeutic Drug Monitoring. 1999;**21**:325-326

[41] DeNofrio D, Loh E, Kao A, Korecka M, et al. Mycophenolic acid concentrations are associated with cardiac allograft rejection. The Journal of Heart and Lung Transplantation. 2000;**19**:1071-1076

[42] Ensom MH, Partovi N, Decarie D, et al. Mycophenolate pharmacokinetics in early period following lung or heart transplantation. The Annals of Pharmacotherapy. 2003; **37**:1761-1767

[43] Eisen H, Ross H. Optimizing the immunosuppressive regimen in heart transplantation. The Journal of Heart and Lung Transplantation. 2004;**23**:S207-S213

[44] Yamani MH, Starling RC, Goormastic M, et al. The impact of routine mycophenolate mofetil drug monitoring on the treatment of cardiac allograft rejection. Transplantation. 2000;**69**:2326-2330

[45] Hesse CJ, Vantrimpont P, van Riemsdijk-van-Overbeeke IC, et al. The value of routine monitoring of mycophenolic acid plasma levels after clinical heart transplantation. Transplantation Proceedings. 2001;**33**:2163-2164

[46] Ratain MJ, Vogelzang NJ. Limited sampling model for vinblastine pharmacokinetics. Cancer Treatment Reports. 1987;**71**:935-939

[47] Ratain MJ, Staubus AE, Schilsky RL, et al. Limited sampling models for amonafide (NSC 308847) pharmacokinetics. Cancer Research. 1988;**48**:4127-4130

[48] Woillard JB, Saint-Marcoux F, Monchaud C, et al. Mycophenolic mofetil optimized pharmacokinetic modelling, and exposure-effect associations in adult heart transplant recipients. Pharmacological Research. 2015;**99**:308-315

[49] Li H, Mager DE, Sandmaier BM, Maloney DG, Bemer MJ, McCune JS. Population pharmacokinetics and dose optimization of mycophenolic acid in HCT recipients receiving oral mycophenolate mofetil. Journal of Clinical Pharmacology. 2013;**53**:393-402

[50] Garg U, Munar A, Frazee C, et al. Determination of mycophenolic acid and mycophenolic acid glucuronide using liquid chromatography tandem mass spectrometry (LC/MS/MS). Current Protocols in Toxicology. 2018;**21**(75):18.21.1-18.21.8

[51] Sheiner LB, Beal SL. Some suggestions for measuring predictive performance. Journal of Pharmacokinetics and Biopharmaceutics. 1981;**9**:503-512

[52] Bland JM, Altman DG. Statistical methods for assessing agreement between two methods of clinical measurement. Lancet. 1986;**1**:307-310

[53] Baraldo M, Isola M, Feruglio MT, et al. Therapeutic mycophenolic acid monitoring by means of limited sampling strategy in orthotopic heart transplant patients. Transplantation Proceedings. 2005;**37**:2240-2243

[54] Baraldo M, Cojutti PG, Isola M, et al. Validation of limited sampling strategy for estimation of mycophenolic acid exposure during the first year after heart transplantation. Transplantation Proceedings. 2009;**41**:4277-4284

[55] Wada K, Takada M, Kotake T, et al. Limited sampling strategy for mycophenolic acid in Japanese heart transplant recipients. Comparison of cyclosporine and tacrolimus treatment. Circulation Journal. 2007;**71**:1022-1028

[56] Kaczmarek I, Bigdeli AK, Vogeser M, et al. Defining algorithms for efficient therapeutic drug monitoring of mycophenolate mofetil in heart transplant recipients. Therapeutic Drug Monitoring. 2008;**30**:419-427

[57] Pawinski T, Kunicki PK, Sobieszczanska-Malek M, et al. A limited sampling strategy for estimating mycophenolic acid area under the curve in adult heart transplant patients treated with concomitant cyclosporine. Journal of Clinical Pharmacy and Therapeutics. 2009;**34**:89-101

[58] Bullingham RES, Nicholls AJ, Kamm BR. Clinical pharmacokinetics of mycophenolate mofetil. Clinical Pharmacokinetics. 1988;**34**:429-455

[59] Dosch AO, Ehlermann P, Koch A, et al. A comparison of measured trough levels and abbreviated AUC estimation by limited sampling strategies for monitoring mycophenolic acid exposure in stable heart transplant patients receiving cyclosporine A-containing and cyclosporine A-free immunosuppressive regimens. Clinical Therapeutics. 2006;**28**:893-905

[60] Ting LS, Partovi N, Levy RD, et al. Performance of limited sampling strategy for predicting mycophenolic acid area under the curve in thoracic transplant recipients. The Journal of Heart and Lung Transplantation. 2008;**27**:325-328

[61] Li P, Shuker N, Hesselink DA, van Schaik RH, Zhang X, van Gelder T. Do Asian renal transplant patients need another mycophenolate mofetil dose compared with Caucasian or African American patients? Transplant International. 2014;**27**:994-1004

[62] Shaw LM, Holt DW, Oellerich M, et al. Current issues in therapeutic drug monitoring of mycophenolic acid: Report of a roundtable discussion. Therapeutic Drug Monitoring. 2001;**23**:305-315